FAST & EZ
CALORIE, FAT,
CARB, FIBER,
& PROTEIN
COUNTER

By Helena Schaar

****

The easiest calorie & complete food counter ever! Alphabetical listings for fast and easy calorie, fat, carbohydrate, fiber, and protein counts. All your favorite foods, fast food restaurants, and beverages. Contains about 3,500 listings. Slim sized to fit in a purse or briefcase.

****

"EZ! Fitness Diet & Exercise Guide" included inside in this book. Here, with a food counter and a fitness guide, you have the only book you need to manage your weight. Here, find the power for a lifetime of total success controlling your weight!

****

FAST & EZ
CALORIE, FAT
CARB, FIBER,
& PROTEIN
COUNTER

By: Helena Schaar

Printed in the United States of America.

This book is dedicated to my son Jasen, & my grandmother Helen, whom I love with all my heart and soul.

About the author:

Helena Schaar is a licensed, registered, healthcare professional with over 15 years of experience. Helena works as a healthcare therapist, college faculty member, and medical writer with over 30 published articles and books. These articles have been approved and accredited by state and national healthcare licensing boards.

Helena and her family live in the sunshine state of Florida. Helena is a lifelong devotee of health and fitness, including calorie counting, good nutrition and plenty of exercise.

FAST & EZ
CALORIE, FAT
CARB, FIBER,
& PROTEIN
COUNTER

By: Helena Schaar

<u>**TABLE OF CONTENTS**</u>   <u>***Page No.**</u>

*E-book online layout may have different page numbers depending on your browser.

INTRODUCTION

Welcome to the FAST & EZ CALORIE, FAT CARB, FIBER, & PROTEIN COUNTER. You now possess the power to control your weight forever. This is a guide to safe, simple, effective methods of managing your weight, while promoting optimal health.

Nutrition experts agree, calories count first in weight management. This book is designed to help you count calories & nutrients accurately, quickly, and easily. Alphabetical listings make locating your foods simple. To improve clarity and speed in locating food choices, this book is divided into 3 sections:

Beverages
Foods
Fast Food Restaurants

This edition is small and slim sized to easily fit into a purse or briefcase. Use it at home while planning meals and carry it wherever you go.

References (2004) for compiling this book are the United States Department of Agriculture (USDA) nutritional database, food manufacturers' nutrient labels, and restaurants printed nutritional data. References for the diet and exercise data are the USDA database and WebMD.com.

Counting calories is a time-honored method for weight management. Nutrition experts agree that <u>calories count first when trying to manage your weight.</u> Other factors can then be addressed, including your activity level, amount of daily exercise, and how you balance your intake of carbohydrates, protein, fat, sodium, and other nutrients.

This book is designed to help make counting calories and other nutrients fast and easy. Precise and accurate alphabetical listings provide for quick calorie counts. Whether you are a pro, or a novice at counting calories and nutrients, you will find this book contains all the information you need. Inside are all the foods you love to eat, prepared the ways most people love to eat them, in the most common serving sizes. This includes the most popular foods, the most common foods, favorite fast food restaurants, brand names, beverages, and alcoholic beverages. About 3,500 listings included.

To use the food counter, simply locate your choice of food or beverage in one of the three alphabetical sections:

Beverages
Foods
Fast Food Restaurants

For the best results, read over the entire book to get an idea of which foods are high in calories and which foods are low in calories. That will help you make smart food choices every time you eat.

Managing your weight is so much easier with the right tools, including a good calorie/nutrient counter, and a simple exercise plan. This food counter includes the EZ! Fitness Diet & Exercise Guide. Here, find all of the essential tools to manage your weight, and shed those unwanted pounds and inches forever. This book gives you the power base for building a lifetime of good health, and the joy of achieving your ideal body weight.

The EZ! Fitness Diet & Exercise Guide also gives you all the information you need to understand calories, healthy dieting, and exercise. The formulas are included to calculate your daily caloric requirements for achieving and maintaining your ideal weight. Calorie expenditure is also covered, including how to burn calories faster. Also information about lifestyle activity factors, and how to increase yours, to burn calories faster. Tips about safe and easy exercise, and plenty of diet tips and secrets. Calorie counting along with a simple exercise routine results in healthy weight management, with long-lasting results.

NOTES:

All listings are medium size or average portion size, unless specifically noted.

"Cooked" means the food is cooked without added fats, sauces, or sugars. This includes boiling, steaming, and heating in a microwave oven.

"Baked" and "Broiled" describe the normal methods of baking and broiling, without oil, or minimal cooking oil for a non-stick surface. No other fats, sauces, or sugars added.

Italics signify registered trademarks for foods.

The data is accurate at the time publication. However, food manufacturers may change their ingredients at any time without notice. Food nutrition labels should also be checked.

ABBREVIATION KEY:

appx	approximately
as prep	prepared as instructed on package, usual method
avg	average size
bev	beverage
cal	calorie
dia	diameter
fl oz	fluid ounce
g	gram(s)
"	inch(es)
Lb	pound
Lg	large
mcg	microgram
med	medium
misc	miscellaneous
mg	milligram(s)
ml	milliliter
oz	ounce
pc	piece
pkg	package
pkt	packet
prep	prepared
sm	small
svg	serving
sq	square
Tbsp	tablespoon
Tr	trace- less than 1 g or mg
tsp	teaspoon
w/	with
w/o	without

Metric Conversion Factors:

Volume	Multiply By	To Find Equivalent
Teaspoons	4.93	Milliliters
Tablespoons	14.79	Milliliters
Fluid ounces	29.57	Milliliters
Cups	0.24	Liters
Gallons	3.79	Liters

Weight	Multiply By	To Find Equivalent
Ounces	28.35	Grams
Pounds	0.45	Kilograms

Approximate Measure Equivalents:

VOLUME

1 Teaspoon = ...5 ml
1 Tablespoon =.....3 Teaspoons =...........15 ml
2 Tablespoons =....1 fl oz = ...30 ml
4 Tablespoons =....¼ Cup = ...2 fl oz = ...59 ml
16 Tablespoons =...1 Cup = ...8 fl oz =.....237 ml
1 Cup =..........½ Pint =.......8 fl oz = ... 237 ml
2 Cups =.........1 Pint =.......16 fl oz = ...474 ml
2 Pints = ...1 Quart =....32 fl oz = ... 946 ml
1 Gallon = ...4 Quarts =..128 fl oz = 3.79 Liters

WEIGHT

1 Ounce = 28 grams
1 Pound = 454 grams

*This table lists approximate metric equivalents for easy reference.

EZ! FITNESS
DIET & EXERCISE GUIDE

By: Helena Schaar

You can be in total control of your weight forever. The facts, tips, and ideas in this guide give you the "need to know" essentials of calories, exercise, and weight management. This guide along with the calorie counter gives you the power and the knowledge to control your weight forever.

These lifetime weight management ideas promote good health. This plan is safe, effective, easy to follow, and fits into any lifestyle. Learn the secrets to weight management, and simple exercise routines that lead to a lifetime of health, well being, and total success in weight control.

Fad diets, crash diets, and starvation diets are not recommended. You may lose weight, however, as soon as you resume your normal eating habits, the weight will return. There are also potential adverse health effects from any type of quick weight loss diet. Starvation diets also lead to a slower metabolism.

For total lifetime control of your weight, it is better to have a diet plan you can easily live with forever; one that does not feel like a diet at all!

Please Note: As with any weight management plan, results may vary for each individual. You should always consult your physician before beginning any new diet or exercise plan; and especially if you have current health problems, or you are pregnant or nursing. This diet plan is offered only as information, for use in maintaining and promoting your good health in cooperation with a physician. In the event that the information presented in this diet plan is used without a physician's approval, the individual using the plan accepts all responsibility. This plan is only intended for normal healthy adults over age 20. Those with underlying health problems may or may not be able to achieve their weight goals, or maintain their weight goals. Always consult your physician first.

This diet plan is very simple: You first choose your ideal body weight. You may know exactly what is right for you, or you can refer to the "Ideal Body Weight" chart. You then calculate the number of daily calories needed to achieve that weight. (Calculations discussed later). You can eat satisfying and well-balanced variety of foods, including all your favorite foods, while making better food choices by counting calories. Read over the Healthy Diet Basics, and the EZ Weight Loss Secrets. If you want to achieve optimal health, you should add a simple exercise routine to your day. Exercise also helps speed up weight loss, and makes lifetime weight management much easier.

When trying to lose weight, several factors come into play that affect the speed of weight loss. This includes:

- How many pounds you are above your ideal weight. Generally, the more you weigh, the faster you will lose weight. Losing 5 to 7 pounds per month is a healthy goal if you are overweight.
- Your commitment to counting and cutting calories and your commitment to get active with exercise.
- Your metabolism. As you age, metabolism naturally slows down. Exercise speeds up the metabolism. Heredity is also a factor; some naturally have a faster metabolism than others.

HEALTHY DIET BASICS

The following is a list of important facts, and healthy tips to keep in mind for smart weight management. These tips will help in achieving and maintaining your ideal weight.

Drink 6 to 8 glasses of water every day. Water helps to cleanse and purify the body, and improves overall health.

Take a multi-vitamin and mineral supplement every day. This helps to assure that you are obtaining all the essential nutrients your body needs.

Eat a variety of foods every day from all of the food groups. Variety and balance in the food groups helps to assure proper nutrition and good health. All types of foods contain varying amounts of vitamins, minerals, and nutrients. The food groups are:

- Bread, grains, oats, wheat, cereal, rice, and pasta. (Good source of carbs and fiber, some protein).

- Fruits and vegetables. (Fruits high in carbs; vegetables contain many nutrients, plus some protein and fiber).

- Dairy products including milk, and cheese. (High in protein and carbs, some are high in fat).

- Meat products including beef, pork, chicken, fish, and eggs. (High in protein, some are high in fat).

- Fats, oils, and sweets. Minimize intake of this food group. (Very high in fat and/or sugar).

The USDA recommendations for variety and balance in daily caloric intake follows:

- 50% to 60% from carbohydrates (carbs)
- 12% to 20% from proteins
- Less than 30% from fats

For example, in an 1800 calorie diet, for a 120 pound adult, the USDA recommends the following daily intake for optimal nutritional health:

Carbohydrates: 250 grams
                (about 55% of total caloric intake)

Protein: 54 grams
                (about 16% of total caloric intake,
                  or 0.45 grams/kg of body weight)

Fat: Less than 58 grams
                (less than 30% of total caloric intake)

Fiber: 23 grams or more. Fiber is found in carbohydrates and is very good for you with multiple health benefits. Fiber is especially good for the heart and colon. Some studies indicate that an increase in fiber with the proper balance of protein increases the metabolism naturally, resulting in faster weight loss, and easier weight management.

Carbohydrates can be classified as simple, such as sugar, or complex. The complex carbs are good for you and contain many nutrients. Carbohydrates also include fiber, which is very good for you. Foods high in complex carbs, such as bread and rice contain many vitamins and minerals. Carbs also contain starch and sugar. Sugar is the so-called "bad carb", high in calories with little nutritional value. You can usually tell a bad carb because it is sweet.

Increased focus has been given to diets that promote very high intake of protein, with very low intake of carbohydrates. This does promote fast weight loss in many people. However, nutrition experts agree that a well balanced diet with higher intake of carbohydrates, less protein, and less fat is safer and healthier. A minor increase in protein intake, with a minor decrease in carbohydrate intake is a better option if considering a high protein/low carb diet. The extremes of almost all protein and fat, with almost no carbohydrate intake can have serious health consequences. Many high protein foods are also high in fat and cholesterol, and some are high in sodium (processed meats). Health problems noted in high protein, high fat, low carb diets include: kidney failure, increased risk of heart disease due to increased cholesterol levels, and increased risk of cancer.

When choosing diets and foods, it is best to stay close to the USDA recommendations for variety, balance, and good nutrition. This will help you achieve lifetime control of your health and weight.

ALL ABOUT CALORIES & WEIGHT

Simply put, if you eat fewer calories, you will lose weight. There are 3500 calories in one pound. For every 3500 calories you cut out of your diet, you will lose one pound of body weight. Calories provide energy. You need calories and the energy derived from calories to live. However, if you consume more calories than your body needs, the result is weight gain. For the safest, healthiest weight loss, you need to maintain the proper caloric intake, balance your food groups, and increase your physical activity level. This leads to good health, good nutrition, and easy to maintain, long lasting results.

You can choose your perfect weight for yourself, or refer to the ideal body weight chart. Then you just determine the number of calories you need per day to achieve that weight. For example: Let's say your ideal perfect weight is 120 pounds, and you have a moderately active lifestyle. You need 1800 calories per day. (See the lifestyle activity levels and factors). No matter what your present weight is, if you begin today to eat 1800 calories per day, and you are a moderately active healthy adult, you will eventually weigh 120 pounds. It's that easy. 1800 calories per day is a satisfying amount of food, it certainly does not seem like a diet to most people. 1800 calories per day leaves plenty of room for good variety, balance, and nutrition. You just need to learn to make smart food choices, and counting calories is the best way.

Read over the calorie counter. Get to know which foods are naturally lower in calories. Reducing your caloric intake, and managing your weight is so much easier once you learn which types of foods are high in calories, and which types of foods are low in calories.

Do you need to spend lots of time counting every calorie?

No. Calorie counting gets easier over time, and after a while it is like second nature. After a few months of using a calorie counter, most people have memorized the approximate calorie counts of favorite foods. While it is true every calorie counts in weight management, it is also true that every bit of activity also counts. It is almost impossible to measure exactly how many calories you burn in a day; you would have to measure calorie expenditure every time you stand up, even every time you move. It is, however, easy to figure approximately how many calories you need, and how many you burn per day with the simple formulas in this book. So, you do not need to spend lots of time counting every calorie. Instead, try rounding and averaging calories to save time, but don't cheat yourself by neglecting to count the majority of your calories.

An easy calorie counting tip is to start the day with 200 calories as a catch-all for any tiny snacks like sugar free candy or gum, diet sodas, other diet beverages, celery or carrot sticks, etc. Then, say for an example, your ideal weight is 120 pounds, and you are a moderately active person. You get to consume 1800 calories per day. Subtract the 200 calorie catch-all, and you have about 1600 calories to divide over 3 meals. After some practice counting calories, you won't even need to write down the daily calorie counts, you will be easily able to keep a daily running total in the back of your mind.

How many calories do you need per day?

There are complicated formulas and expensive tests to determine your caloric requirements based on basal metabolism. A very simple rule of thumb is to choose your ideal weight (the weight you consider perfect for yourself) and multiply by 15 to determine your daily caloric requirements. This formula is correct for moderately active, healthy adults over age 20. The activity levels and factors are discussed in the next section.

If you are extremely active, your caloric requirements will be higher. If you are sedentary, your caloric requirements will be lower.

(Notes: Caloric requirements decrease with age as the metabolism slows down. Caloric requirements can be significantly increased during any illness.)

FORMULA FOR CALCULATING DAILY CALORIES NEEDED:

Multiply your ideal body weight by your activity factor to determine daily caloric requirements.

Example: A moderately active adult who wants to weigh 120 pounds, needs 1800 calories per day.

$$120 \times 15 = 1800$$

CALORIE EXPENDITURE & EXERCISE

Calorie expenditure describes the process of the body utilizing or burning calories for energy. Different activities burn calories at different levels. You can measure your overall lifestyle activity level and the factors by using this chart. You can then make adjustments to your activity level, and add exercises that help burn calories faster.

LIFESTYLE ACTIVITY LEVELS & FACTORS

Sedentary Lifestyle   (Factor = 12)
   Sitting most of the day, no formal exercise program.

Moderately Active Lifestyle   (Factor = 15)
   Performs regular moderately strenuous exercise program at least 3 times per week for at least 20 minutes per session. Good amount of walking and activity in normal daily routine.

Vigorously Active Lifestyle   (Factor = 18)
   Extremely active. Performs regular strenuous exercise at least 5 times per week for at least 30 minutes per session. Exercise program includes running or jogging at fast pace, high impact aerobic type exercise, or equally strenuous exercise. Daily routine and/or job include lots of physical activity.

If you fall somewhere in the middle, your activity factor will fall somewhere in the middle of these activity factors.

Tip: Every time you perform a physical activity or exercise, you are burning more calories than if you are sitting. So a key to losing weight faster, is to GET ACTIVE! Take the stairs whenever possible, take a walk after eating, find an exercise or activity you enjoy, and add it to your daily routine. Adding a simple exercise like walking, biking, or swimming to your daily routine, for 20 minutes per day, 3 to 5 days per week will help to speed up weight loss, increase muscle tone, and increase your energy level.

Which exercises burn more calories?

Simply, the more strenuous the exercise, the more calories you burn. You can also gauge how vigorous the exercise is by checking your heart rate.

Weight training/weightlifting is a little different than other exercises. You may or may not increase you heart rate as much as with other exercises, but you are still doing yourself a world of good. Weight training is very effective at toning muscles and increasing lean muscle mass. This means you will have less fat and more muscle on your body. Muscle also weighs more than fat, so you will need more calories per day to maintain your weight. You can also achieve your ideal physique by adjusting the amount of weights you train with, and the number of repetitions you perform. You can choose to be anywhere from slim and well toned to very muscular. Most women prefer the slim and well-toned look. To achieve that, use light weights and more repetitions. Two to five pound weights that can be held in each hand are ideal. Lift them over your head in slow repetitions for 10 minutes, and work your way up to 20 minutes. Perform this exercise 3 times per week. This can be combined with riding an indoor stationary bike to save time, and get an all over workout.

An exercise is classified as aerobic if you can achieve and maintain your maximum heart rate range for at least 20 minutes, and preferably 30 minutes. Aerobic exercise provides a <u>multitude</u> of health benefits. This includes:

- Increased energy levels
- Faster weight loss
- Improved overall health
- Lower blood pressure and lower resting heart rate (This is a long-term beneficial aspect of aerobic exercise).

Before beginning an exercise, check your normal resting heart rate. The normal for an adult is 60 to 100 beats per minute, with 80 being the average normal value. Count the heartbeat for 15 seconds and multiply by 4 to calculate beats per minute. Then check your heart rate periodically while performing an exercise, to be sure you are maintaining the aerobic level.

<u>Using heart rate to calculate aerobic exercise level:</u>

Your target heart rate while exercising is calculated as follows:

220 (minus your age) x (75% to 85%)

Example: for a 35 year old female:
220 – 35 = 185 x 75% = 139

In this example, the 35 year old female can gauge the exercise activity level by her heart rate increase from a resting heart rate of 80 to the aerobic exercise heart rate of 139. The heart rate should be checked periodically to gauge the aerobic level. Note: If your heart rate is much higher than calculated in the formula, you should stop exercising, and consult your physician before restarting aerobic exercise. Using 85% in the formula above instead of 75% is the <u>maximum</u> heart rate you should achieve. Also, any illness including a fever can increase heart rate, so the heart rates given here are for normal healthy adults only. Always check with your doctor before beginning any exercise program.

Calorie expenditure chart*

Calorie expenditure increases with more strenuous exercise and activity. This chart reveals some common activities and the number of calories burned per hour during these activities.

*Calories burned per hour in this example are approximate values for a normal healthy adult female weighing 130 pounds, or a normal, healthy adult male weighing 165 pounds.

<u>Activity/Exercise</u>	<u>*Calories burned per hour</u>	
	<u>Female</u>	<u>Male</u>
<u>Sitting quietly</u>	60	80
<u>Standing still</u>	75	100

<u>Light activity/exercise</u>
  Cleaning the house
  Walking slowly/strolling
  Playing golf
	210	250

<u>Moderate activity/exercise</u>
  Bicycling at 6 mph
  Fast power walking at 3.5 mph
  Swimming at a moderate pace
  Low/Moderate impact aerobics
  Dancing at moderate pace
  Moderate weight training
  Playing basketball or tennis
	330	410

Strenuous activity/exercise	**620**	**800**

High impact aerobics
Swimming very fast
Jogging/running at 8 mph or faster
Jumping rope very fast
Stair stepping
Cross country skiing

ACTIVITY/EXERCISE TIPS:

Choose an activity you enjoy, and perform it regularly for 20 minutes per day at least three days per week. This will promote faster weight loss, easier weight management, improved overall health, and improved sense of well being.

This exercise can be as simple as walking. You can walk outside and get the added benefit of fresh air, or if the weather is poor, you can simulate a walk inside while watching your favorite television program, or catching up on the news. You should walk at a fast pace, but one that is comfortable to you. Don't walk so fast that you get short of breath. Your stamina and endurance will increase the longer you continue. If you are walking inside, be sure to really lift your feet off the floor. Whether indoors or outdoors, you should swing your arms back and forth, or continuously lift them over your head as if reaching for the sky. This provides for all-over muscle toning. If you want to tone up your arm muscles faster, and burn lots of extra calories, you can hold weights in your hands while you walk. Another option is to strap weights to your ankles. Two or three pound weights are ideal, very easy to find, and very inexpensive.

Bicycling is also a very enjoyable exercise for many. This can be done indoors on a stationary bike or outdoors in the fresh air. Indoor bikes should have tension controls so you can adjust your calorie expenditure based on endurance. Here again, weights can be used to burn lots of extra calories and tone the arms. Two or three pound weights are ideal. Hold them in your hands and lift upward in repetitions. If biking outdoors, find routes with hills, if possible, for maximum calorie expenditure.

Once you have mastered one exercise, you can step up to a higher activity level exercise. Read over the list to see which ones burn more calories, and find one you truly enjoy. Once you have achieved your ideal weight, continue the exercise routine, or even step up a level, to maintain your optimal good health and your ideal weight.

EZ! Weight Loss Secrets

Try one, two, or all of these tips for easy weight loss. Step on the scale a week later, or a month later and be amazed at the results! Be sure to also follow the Healthy Diet Basics outlined earlier.

- Many of your favorite foods come in low calorie, light, sugar free, low fat, and fat free versions that are almost equal in taste. Try it, you might like it! The result of switching to the low calorie versions of foods and drinks is fast and easy weight loss. Try it for ¼, or ½, or more of the foods and beverages you consume, and be amazed at the results. Of course, it is impractical to do this for all of your foods. Everyone wants to enjoy special foods and drinks for holidays, special occasions, eating out with friends, and just because it's good to treat yourself. Remember that a little bit of almost everything is good for you, a lot of almost anything is bad for you.

- After the special occasions, you can easily get right back into the pattern of healthy eating.

- By switching to the sugar free or calorie-free version of most of your beverages, you can cut your daily caloric intake considerably; even up to 800 calories per day, with very little effort.

- When you choose foods in the low calorie, light, sugar free, low fat, or fat free versions, you save anywhere from 10% to 90% of the calories for that dish. For example, a rice dish made with 1 tablespoon of regular butter has 250 calories. If you use fat free margarine instead of regular butter, the total calories are about 150, saving you 100 calories. A salad with 2 tablespoons of fat free dressing instead of regular dressing saves you about 120 calories.

- Prepare your food without adding cooking oil that has 120 calories per tablespoon. Try baking, broiling, or grilling with a non-stick cooking spray that has zero calories.

- With sugar free fruit flavored beverages like *Crystal Light* or *Kool Aid*, you can save about 100 calories per cup over regular fruit flavored beverages. These come in many varieties and are excellent thirst quenchers. With soft drinks, you can reduce the calories from about 150 to zero by switching to a diet version of the soda.

- For between meal snacks, try anything low calorie, and low fat. Some examples are sugar free gum and candy, vegetables with fat free dip, carrot sticks, and any diet beverage. With just a small snack you will easily be able to curb your cravings for an hour or two until your next meal.

- Choose foods that are low in fat, salt, and sugar, these foods are naturally lower in calories and promote weight loss. Also avoid high sodium foods to avoid water retention weight gain.

- Add a little physical activity at least three to five days per week. Read the "All About Calories" topic which includes calorie expenditure charts as related to exercise. To begin, choose a simple and pleasant exercise such as walking, swimming, or riding a bicycle. Just 20 minutes per day, a few days per week, can dramatically accelerate your weight loss, increase energy levels, and improve your overall sense of well being. Your brain releases endorphins when you exercise. Endorphins are chemicals that make you feel good, and the feeling can last for many hours after you finish exercising. Many people who exercise regularly say they feel energized all day long. Let the endorphins flow!

Ideal Body Weight Chart

The following chart is to help you calculate your ideal body weight. This chart is for adults age 20 and over. The data is compiled from various medical and health journals. There is a wide range of what is considered to be the "ideal" body weight. This chart lists weights for a medium frame, with one to two pounds of clothing on. Heights listed are without shoes. You should only weigh yourself in the morning, before eating or drinking anything. This is the best way to track the trend of your weight loss, since your weight can fluctuate throughout the day, especially after eating a meal. You should use this chart only as an estimated guide to your ideal weight.

FEMALE:

Height (Feet' Inches")	Ideal Body Weight (in Pounds)
5'0"	100 – 110
5'1"	102 – 112
5'2"	105 – 118
5'3"	108 – 122
5'4"	110 – 125
5"5"	114 – 130
5'6"	116 – 136
5'7"	120 – 140
5'8"	125 – 145
5'10"	130 – 155

MALE:

Height (Feet'Inches")	Ideal Body Weight (in Pounds)
5'4"	125 – 140
5'6"	135 – 155
5'8"	145 – 165
5'10"	160 – 175
6'0"	170 – 185
6'2"	180 – 195

****

Good wishes and the best of health to you!

****

BEVERAGES

BEVERAGE: (See Food and Fast Food Restaurants listed separately)	Serving Size	Cal- ories	Fat (g)	Carb (g)	Fi- ber (g)	Pro- tein (g)
Amaretto, 53 proof	1.5 fl oz	175	Tr	24	0	Tr
Apple Juice	8 fl oz	115	Tr	29	Tr	Tr
Apple-Cranberry Juice	8 fl oz	115	Tr	29	Tr	Tr
Apple-Grape Juice	8 fl oz	130	Tr	31	Tr	Tr
Apple-Raspberry Juice	8 fl oz	120	Tr	30	Tr	Tr
Apricot Nectar	8 fl oz	140	Tr	36	Tr	Tr
Beer	...	.	.	.	.	.
Regular Beer	12 fl oz	150	0	13	1	1
Light Beer	12 fl oz	100	0	6	0	1
Dark beer	12 fl oz	160	0	14	Tr	1
Draft beer, regular	12 fl oz	150	0	13	Tr	1
Draft beer, light	12 fl oz	100	0	6	0	1
Dry beer	12 fl oz	130	0	8	Tr	1
Malt beer	12 fl oz	160	0	10	Tr	1
Bloody Mary	5 fl oz	150	Tr	5	Tr	1
Bourbon	...	...	.	.	.	.
80 proof	1.5 fl oz	95	0	0	0	0
86 proof	1.5 fl oz	105	0	Tr	0	0
90 proof	1.5 fl oz	110	0	Tr	0	0
Brandy	...	...	.	.	.	.
80 proof	1.5 fl oz	95	0	0	0	0
86 proof	1.5 fl oz	105	0	Tr	0	0
90 proof	1.5 fl oz	110	0	Tr	0	0
Flavored, 60 proof, (Apricot Blackberry, Cherry, or Coffee)	... 1.5 fl oz	... 180	. Tr.	. 24	. 0	. Tr
Capri Sun juice drink	8 fl oz	122	Tr	31	Tr	Tr
Carbonated Beverages- see Soda	...	...	.	.	.	.
Carrot Juice	8 fl oz	95	Tr	22	2	2
Club Soda	12 fl oz	0	0	0	0	0
Cocoa / Chocolate Beverage, Hot	...	...	.	.	.	.
Regular, as prep	6 fl oz	170	7	23	1	7
Diet or sugarfree, as prep	6 fl oz	35	0	5	Tr	3
COFFEE	...	...	.	.	.	.
Brewed coffee, regular or decaf	6 fl oz	4	0	1	0	Tr
Instant coffee, regular or decaf	6 fl oz	4	0	1	0	Tr
Café Amaretto	6 fl oz	70	2	6	0	7

BEVERAGE: (See Food and Fast Food Restaurants listed separately)	Serving Size	Cal-ories	Fat (g)	Carb (g)	Fi-ber (g)	Pro-tein (g)
Café Latte	6 fl oz	115	6	10	0	6
Café Vienna	6 fl oz	70	2	6	0	7
Cappuccino	6 fl oz	65	3	6	0	3
Espresso	2 fl oz	5	Tr	1	0	Tr
French Vanilla Café	6 fl oz	70	2	6	0	7
French Vanilla, sugarfree	6 fl oz	20	Tr	4	0	Tr
Hazelnut Belgian Cafe	6 fl oz	75	2	7	0	7
Swiss Mocha coffee	6 fl oz	75	1	8	Tr	9
Swiss Mocha coffee, sugarfree	6 fl oz	20	Tr	4	0	Tr
Viennese Chocolate coffee	6 fl oz	75	1	8	Tr	9
Coffee Cream – see Creamer	...	...	.	.	.	.
Coffee Liqueur, 53 proof	1.5 fl oz	175	Tr	24	0	Tr
Coke - see Soda	...	...	.	.	.	.
Cola - see Soda	...	...	.	.	.	.
Cranapple Drink	8 fl oz	170	0	43	Tr	0
Cranberry Juice Cocktail	8 fl oz	145	Tr	36	Tr	0
Cranberry-Grape Drink	8 fl oz	145	Tr	34	Tr	Tr
Creamer	.	.	.	.	.	.
Half & Half (cream & milk)	1 Tbsp	20	2	1	0	1
Half & Half (cream & milk)	1 cup	315	28	10	0	7
Liquid creamer Coffee-Mate	1 Tbsp	20	1	2	0	Tr
Powdered creamer Coffee-Mate	1 tsp	10	Tr	2	0	Tr
Crème de Menthe	1 fl oz	125	0	14	0	0
Crystal Light, all flavors	8 fl oz	5	0	0	0	0
Daiquiri, strawberry	4 fl oz	225	Tr	8	Tr	Tr
Diet Cola	12 fl oz	0	0	0	0	0
Diet or sugarfree Kool Aid	8 fl oz	5	0	1	Tr	0
Diet Soda	12 fl oz	0	0	0	0	0
Eggnog, plain	1 cup	345	19	34	0	10
Fruit Drink (5% to 10% juice)	...	...	.	.	.	.
Cherry, Grape, Orange,	...	...	.	.	.	.
or Strawberry	...	...	.	.	.	.
Regular	8 fl oz	135	0	32	Tr	0
Sugarfree	8 fl oz	5	0	1	Tr	0
Fruit Punch (10% Juice)	...	...	.	.	.	.
Regular	8 fl oz	130	0	31	Tr	0
Sugarfree	8 fl oz	5	0	1	Tr	0
Gatorade	8 fl oz	50	0	14	0	0
Gin	...	...	.	.	.	.
80 proof	1.5 fl oz	95	0	0	0	0

BEVERAGE: (See Food and Fast Food Restaurants listed separately)	Serving Size	Cal- ories	Fat (g)	Carb (g)	Fi- ber (g)	Pro- tein (g)
86 proof	1.5 fl oz	105	0	Tr	0	0
90 proof	1.5 fl oz	110	0	Tr	0	0
Grape Juice	...	...	.	.	.	.
Canned or bottled, sweetened	8 fl oz	155	Tr	38	Tr	1
Frozen concentrate, sweetened,	.	.	.	.	.	.
as prep w/ water	8 fl oz	130	Tr	32	Tr	Tr
Unsweetened grape juice	8 fl oz	120	Tr	30	Tr	Tr
Grapefruit Juice	...	...	.	.	.	.
Fresh, squeezed, unsweetened	8 fl oz	95	Tr	22	Tr	1
Fresh, squeezed, sugar sweetened	8 fl oz	115	Tr	28	Tr	1
Fresh, squeezed, w/ aspartame	8 fl oz	95	Tr	22	Tr	1
Canned, unsweetened	8 fl oz	95	Tr	22	Tr	1
Canned, sugar sweetened	8 fl oz	115	Tr	28	Tr	1
Frozen concentrate, unsweetened,	...	.	.	.	.	.
as prep w/ water	8 fl oz	100	Tr	24	Tr	1
Half & Half – see Creamer	...	...	.	.	.	.
Hawaiian Punch	...	...	.	.	.	.
Regular	8 fl oz	120	0	30	Tr	0
Sugarfree	8 fl oz	15	0	4	Tr	0
Hot Cocoa/Chocolate – see	...	...	.	.	.	.
Cocoa	...	...	.	.	.	.
Juice – see specific listings	...	...	.	.	.	.
Kool Aid	...	...	.	.	.	.
Sugar sweetened	8 fl oz	60	0	16	Tr	0
Sugarfree	8 fl oz	5	0	1	Tr	0
Unsweetened Packet	1 pkt	0	0	0	0	0
Lemon Juice	...	...	.	.	.	.
Fresh, squeezed, unsweetened	1 Tbsp	4	Tr	1	Tr	Tr
Canned or bottled, unsweetened	1 Tbsp	3	Tr	1	Tr	Tr
Canned or bottled, unsweetened	1 cup	50	1	16	1	1
Lemonade	...	...	.	.	.	.
Sugar Sweetened	8 fl oz	100	0	25	Tr	0
Sugarfree	8 fl oz	5	0	1	Tr	0
Lime Juice	...	...	.	.	.	.
Fresh or bottled, unsweetened	1 Tbsp	3	Tr	1	Tr	Tr
Fresh or bottled, unsweetened	1 cup	52	1	16	1	1
Limeade	...	...	.	.	.	.
Sugar sweetened	8 fl oz	100	0	25	Tr	0
Sugarfree	8 fl oz	5	0	1	Tr	0
Liqueur, 53 proof	...	...	.	.	.	.
Coffee or Fruit Flavored	1.5 fl oz	175	Tr	24	0	Tr

BEVERAGE: (See Food and Fast Food Restaurants listed separately)	Serving Size	Cal-ories	Fat (g)	Carb (g)	Fi-ber (g)	Pro-tein (g)
Mai Tai	5 fl oz	280	Tr	28	1	1
Margarita	5 fl oz	150	0	10	Tr	0
Martini	2.5 fl oz	155	0	0	0	0
Milk	...	...	.	.	.	.
White Milk	...	...	.	.	.	.
Whole milk, 3.3% fat	8 fl oz	150	8	11	0	8
Reduced fat milk, 2% fat	8 fl oz	120	5	12	0	8
Lowfat milk, 1% fat	8 fl oz	102	3	12	0	8
Nonfat milk, (Skim milk)	8 fl oz	85	Tr	12	0	8
Nonfat instant, as prep w/water	8 fl oz	80	0	12	0	8
Nonfat instant, dry powder only	1 cup	240	0	36	0	24
Chocolate Milk	...	...	.	.	.	.
Whole chocolate milk	8 fl oz	210	8	26	2	8
Reduced fat chocolate milk, 2%	8 fl oz	180	5	26	1	8
Lowfat chocolate milk, 1%	8 fl oz	160	3	26	1	8
Misc Milk Products	...	...	.	.	.	.
Buttermilk	1 cup	100	2	12	0	8
Condensed, sweetened	1 cup	980	27	166	0	24
Evaporated whole milk	1 cup	340	19	25	0	17
Evaporated skim milk	1 cup	200	1	29	0	19
Malted milk, chocolate	1 cup	225	9	29	Tr	9
Malted milk, natural	1 cup	230	9	28	0	10
Soy milk	1 cup	81	5	4	3	7
Milk Shake – see Shake	...	...	.	.	.	.
Miso	1 cup	567	17	77	15	32
Nesquik, Chocolate, as prep	8 fl oz	210	5	33	1	7
Orange Juice	...	...	.	.	.	.
Fresh, squeezed, unsweetened	8 fl oz	112	Tr	26	1	2
Canned or bottled, unsweetened	8 fl oz	110	Tr	25	1	2
Frozen concentrate, as prep	8 fl oz	112	Tr	26	1	2
Peach Nectar	8 fl oz	135	0	34	Tr	1
Pear Nectar	8 fl oz	150	0	39	Tr	0
Pepsi – see Soda	...	...	.	.	.	.
Pina Colada	4.5 fl oz	260	3	40	1	1
Pineapple Grapefruit Juice	8 fl oz	120	Tr	29	Tr	1
Pineapple Juice	8 fl oz	140	Tr	34	1	1
Pineapple Orange Juice	8 fl oz	125	0	30	Tr	3
Prune Juice	8 fl oz	182	Tr	45	3	2
Root Beer	...	...	.	.	.	.
Regular	12 fl oz	170	0	47	0	0

BEVERAGE: (See Food and Fast Food Restaurants listed separately)	Serving Size	Cal- ories	Fat (g)	Carb (g)	Fi- ber (g)	Pro- tein (g)
Diet or sugarfree	12 fl oz	0	0	0	0	0
Rum	...	...	.	.	.	.
80 proof	1.5 fl oz	95	0	0	0	0
86 proof	1.5 fl oz	105	0	Tr	0	0
90 proof	1.5 fl oz	110	0	Tr	0	0
Scotch	...	...	.	.	.	.
80 proof	1.5 fl oz	95	0	0	0	0
86 proof	1.5 fl oz	105	0	Tr	0	0
90 proof	1.5 fl oz	110	0	Tr	0	0
Screwdriver	7 fl oz	160	Tr	17	1	Tr
Shake	...	...	.	.	.	.
Regular milk shake	...	...	.	.	.	.
Chocolate	11 oz	360	8	63	1	9
Peach	11 oz	380	4	75	1	10
Strawberry	11 oz	395	4	80	1	11
Vanilla	11 0z	350	9	56	0	12
Low Carb shake	...	...	.	.	.	.
Atkins chocolate shake	11 oz	170	9	5	3	20
Atkins vanilla shake	11 oz	170	9	4	2	20
Soda / Cola / Soft Drink	...	...	.	.	.	.
(Carbonated Beverages)	...	...	.	.	.	.
Club Soda	12 fl oz	0	0	0	0	0
Cherry Cola, regular	12 fl oz	155	0	40	0	0
Cherry Cola, diet	12 fl oz	0	0	0	0	0
Coca Cola, Coke regular	12 fl oz	140	0	39	0	0
Coke, diet	12 fl oz	0	0	0	0	0
Cola	12 fl oz	150	0	40	0	0
Diet Cola	12 fl oz	0	0	0	0	0
Dr Pepper, regular	12 fl oz	150	0	40	0	0
Dr Pepper, diet	12 fl oz	0	0	0	0	0
Ginger Ale, regular	12 fl oz	125	0	32	0	0
Ginger Ale, diet	12 fl oz	0	0	0	0	0
Grape Soda, regular	12 fl oz	155	0	40	0	0
Grape Soda, diet	12 fl oz	0	0	0	0	0
Lemon Lime Soda, regular	12 fl oz	145	0	36	0	0
Lemon Lime Soda, diet	12 fl oz	0	0	0	0	0
Mountain Dew, regular	12 fl oz	170	0	46	0	0
Mountain Dew, diet	12 fl oz	0	0	0	0	0
Mr. Pibb, regular	12 fl oz	146	0	39	0	0
Mr. Pibb, diet	12 fl oz	0	0	0	0	0
Orange Soda, regular	12 fl oz	175	0	45	0	0

BEVERAGE: (See Food and Fast Food Restaurants listed separately)	Serving Size	Cal-ories	Fat (g)	Carb (g)	Fi-ber (g)	Pro-tein (g)
Orange Soda, diet	12 fl oz	0	0	0	0	0
Pepsi, regular	12 fl oz	150	0	41	0	0
Pepsi, diet	12 fl oz	0	0	0	0	0
RC Cola, regular	12 fl oz	160	0	43	0	0
RC Cola, diet	12 fl oz	0	0	0	0	0
Root Beer, Regular	12 fl oz	170	0	44	0	0
Root Beer, Diet	12 fl oz	0	0	0	0	0
Seven Up, regular	12 fl oz	150	0	39	0	0
Seven Up, diet	12 fl oz	0	0	0	0	0
Sprite, regular	12 fl oz	150	0	39	0	0
Sprite, diet	12 fl oz	0	0	0	0	0
Tab	12 fl oz	1	0	0	0	0
Soft Drinks – see Soda	...	...	.	.	.	.
Sport Drink	12 fl oz	75	0	18	0	0
Sugarfree Beverage (Also see specific listings)	... ...	. .	. .	. .	. .	. .
Sugarfree Soda	12 fl oz	0	0	0	0	0
Sugarfree Kool Aid	8 fl oz	5	0	1	Tr	0
Sunny Delight, Citrus Punch	8 fl oz	125	0	31	Tr	0
Tang, regular	8 fl oz	115	0	29	Tr	0
Tang, sugarfree	8 fl oz	5	0	Tr	Tr	0
Tea, Hot or Iced	...	...	.	.	.	.
Regular, unsweetened	8 fl oz	2	0	1	0	0
Regular, sugar sweetened	8 fl oz	90	0	22	0	0
Regular, aspartame sweetened	8 fl oz	4	0	1	0	0
Chamomile tea, unsweetened	8 fl oz	2	0	Tr	0	0
Chamomile tea, sugar sweetened	8 fl oz	90	0	21	0	0
Misc Types of Tea, Blends,	...	...	.	.	.	.
Black, Chinese, Orange Pekoe	...	...	.	.	.	.
Unsweetened	8 fl oz	2	0	Tr	0	0
Sugar sweetened	8 fl oz	90	0	22	0	0
Sweetened w/aspartame	8 fl oz	4	0	1	0	0
Tequila	1.5 fl oz	100	0	0	0	0
Tequila Sunrise	5.5 fl oz	190	0	15	1	1
Tomato Juice	8 fl oz	41	Tr	10	1	2
V 8 Vegetable Juice, 1 Lg can	11 fl oz	70	0	15	2	2
Vegetable Juice	8 fl oz	46	Tr	11	2	2
Vodka	...	...	.	.	.	.
80 proof	1.5 fl oz	95	0	0	0	0
86 proof	1.5 fl oz	105	0	Tr	0	0
90 proof	1.5 fl oz	110	0	Tr	0	0

BEVERAGE: (See Food and Fast Food Restaurants listed separately)	Serving Size	Cal- ories	Fat (g)	Carb (g)	Fi- ber (g)	Pro- tein (g)
Water	8 fl oz	0	0	0	0	0
Whiskey	...	...	.	.	.	.
80 proof	1.5 fl oz	95	0	0	0	0
86 proof	1.5 fl oz	105	0	Tr	0	0
90 proof	1.5 fl oz	110	0	Tr	0	0
Wine	...	...	.	.	.	.
Dessert Wine, Dry	4 fl oz	150	0	5	0	Tr
Dessert Wine, Sweet	4 fl oz	180	0	14	0	Tr
Red Wine (table wine)	4 fl oz	85	0	2	0	Tr
Rosè Wine	4 fl oz	85	0	1	0	Tr
White Wine (table wine)	4 fl oz	80	0	1	0	Tr
White Zinfandel	4 fl oz	85	0	1	0	Tr
Wine Cooler	5.5 fl oz	100	0	11	0	Tr
Wine Spritzer	5.5 fl oz	60	0	1	0	Tr

FOODS

FOOD: (See Beverages & Fast Food Restaurants listed separately)	Serving Size	Cal-ories	Fat (g)	Carb (g)	Fi-ber (g)	Pro-tein (g)
Accent Seasoning	¼ tsp	Tr	0	0	0	0
Alfalfa sprouts, fresh	1 cup	10	Tr	1	Tr	1
Almonds – see Nuts	...	...	.	.	.	.
Anchovy – see Fish	...	...	.	.	.	.
Anise Seed	1 Tbsp	28	1	3	1	1
Apple	...	...	.	.	.	.
Fresh, unpeeled, avg 2 ¾" dia	1	80	Tr	21	4	Tr
Fresh, peeled, sliced	1 cup	65	Tr	16	2	Tr
Dried	5 rings	80	Tr	21	3	Tr
Apple Butter	1 Tbsp	30	0	7	Tr	Tr
Apple Pie Filling	2 oz can	85	11	17	1	1
	1 Tbsp	40	1	8	1	Tr
Applesauce	...	...	.	.	.	.
Sweetened	½ cup	97	Tr	25	2	Tr
Unsweetened	½ cup	52	Tr	14	2	Tr
Apricot	...	...	.	.	.	.
Fresh, medium size, 1.3 oz	1	17	Tr	4	1	Tr
Canned, in heavy syrup	1 cup	215	Tr	55	4	1
Canned, in juice	1 cup	115	Tr	30	4	2
Dried, halves	10 hlvs	85	Tr	22	3	1
Artichoke, Globe or French	...	...	.	.	.	.
Fresh, medium size, cooked	1	60	Tr	13	7	4
Fresh, cooked, drained	1 cup	84	Tr	19	9	6
Jerusalem artichoke, raw, sliced	1 cup	114	Tr	26	2	3
Arugula, raw	½ cup	3	0	Tr	Tr	Tr
Asparagus, cooked	...	.	.	.	.	.
Fresh, medium size spears	4 spears	14	Tr	3	1	2
Fresh, chopped pieces	1 cup	43	1	8	3	5
Frozen, spears	4 spears	17	Tr	3	1	2
Frozen, chopped pieces	1 cup	50	1	9	3	5
Canned, 5" spears	4 spears	14	Tr	2	1	2
Canned, chopped pieces	1 cup	46	2	6	4	5
Aspartame Sweetener	1 pkt	0	0	Tr	0	0
Avocado	...	...	.	.	.	.
California, 1/5 of whole	1 oz	50	5	2	1	1
Florida, 1/10 of whole	1 oz	30	3	3	1	Tr
Bacon – see Pork	...	...	.	.	.	.

FOOD: (See Beverages & Fast Food Restaurants listed separately)	Serving Size	Cal- ories	Fat (g)	Carb (g)	Fi- ber (g)	Pro- tein (g)
Bacon Bits	1 Tbsp	31	2	2	1	2
Bagel, 3 ½" dia	...	...	.	.	.	.
Plain	1	150	1	34	2	4
Cinnamon raisin	1	170	1	36	2	5
Egg	1	160	1	34	2	5
Multigrain	1	150	1	33	3	5
Baking Powder	1 tsp	2	0	1	Tr	0
Baking Soda	1 tsp	0	0	0	0	0
Bamboo Shoots, cooked	1 cup	25	1	4	2	2
Banana	...	...	.	.	.	.
Fresh, 7" long	1	110	1	28	3	1
Fresh, sliced	1 cup	140	1	35	4	2
Banana Split	1	510	12	96	4	8
Barley	...	...	.	.	.	.
Pearled, cooked	1 cup	195	1	44	6	4
Pearled, uncooked	1 cup	705	2	155	31	20
Basil, dried spice	½ tsp	3	0	Tr	Tr	Tr
Bean Sprouts (mung), cooked	1 cup	30	Tr	5	2	3
BEANS	...	...	.	.	.	.
Plain Beans, cooked w/o fats	...	...	.	.	.	.
Black beans	½ cup	115	1	21	8	7
Great Northern beans	½ cup	105	1	19	6	7
Green beans	½ cup	22	Tr	5	3	1
Kidney, Red beans	½ cup	112	1	20	7	7
Lima, large beans	½ cup	100	1	17	8	7
Lima, baby lima beans	½ cup	95	1	17	10	6
Pinto beans	½ cup	117	1	22	7	7
Soybeans	½ cup	135	6	10	5	12
Wax beans	½ cup	25	Tr	5	3	1
White beans	½ cup	150	1	28	6	9
Yellow beans	½ cup	22	Tr	5	3	1
Misc Bean Dishes, as prep	...	...	.	.	.	.
Baked beans, plain or vegetarian	½ cup	118	1	26	6	6
Baked beans, BBQ style	½ cup	180	3	32	7	5
Baked beans w/frankfurters	½ cup	185	8	20	9	9
Baked beans w/tomato sauce	½ cup	125	2	25	6	7
Baked beans w/sweet sauce	½ cup	140	2	27	7	7
Beans w/ pork	½ cup	130	2	24	6	5
Black beans w/ rice	½ cup	150	5	23	5	4
Green bean casserole	½ cup	140	2	13	5	3
Green beans w/almonds	½ cup	60	2	8	4	3

FOOD: (See Beverages & Fast Food Restaurants listed separately)	Serving Size	Cal-ories	Fat (g)	Carb (g)	Fi-ber (g)	Pro-tein (g)
Red beans & rice	½ cup	130	2	23	6	4
Refried beans	½ cup	118	2	20	7	7
BEEF	...	...	.	.	.	.
(Weights for meat w/o bones)	...	...	.	.	.	.
(Meats as prep: braised, broiled,	...	...	.	.	.	.
grilled, simmered, or roasted)	...	...	.	.	.	.
Bottom Round, lean & fat	3 oz	235	14	0	0	24
lean only	3 oz	180	7	0	0	27
Brisket	3 oz	250	17	0	0	23
Chuck Blade, lean & fat	3 oz	295	22	0	0	23
lean only	3 oz	215	11	0	0	26
Corned Beef, canned	3 oz	215	13	0	0	23
Dried Beef, chipped	1 oz	45	1	Tr	0	8
Eye of Round, lean & fat	3 oz	195	11	0	0	23
lean only	3 oz	145	4	0	0	25
Flank Steak	3 oz	225	14	0	0	23
Ground Beef /	...	...	.	.	.	.
Hamburger meat, regular	3 oz	250	18	0	0	20
lean, 79%	3 oz	230	16	0	0	21
extra lean, 83%	3 oz	220	14	0	0	22
Liver of beef, fried	3 oz	185	7	7	0	23
Pastrami	2 oz	90	4	2	Tr	12
Porterhouse Steak	3.5 oz	325	26	0	0	22
Pot Roast, Chuck	3.5 oz	345	26	0	0	27
Prime Ribs	3.5 oz	400	34	0	0	23
Rib Roast, lean & fat	3 oz	305	25	0	0	19
lean only	3 oz	195	11	0	0	23
Roast Beef	3.5 oz	290	20	0	0	25
Short Ribs	3.5 oz	470	42	0	0	22
Sirloin Steak, lean & fat	3 oz	220	13	0	0	24
lean only	3 oz	165	6	0	0	26
T-bone Steak, lean & fat	3.5 oz	310	23	0	0	23
lean only	3.5 oz	250	16	0	0	25
Tenderloin Steak/ Top Loin	3.5 oz	305	22	0	0	25
Top Round	3.5 oz	215	9	0	0	32
(Other Beef Products, see:	...	...	.	.	.	.
Bologna, Hot Dog, Salami,	...	...	.	.	.	.
Sausage & specific entrées)	...	...	.	.	.	.
Beef & Macaroni	...	...	.	.	.	.
Healthy Choice, frozen	1 pkg	210	2	33	5	14
Beef Burgundy, Le Menu entrée	1 meal	315	19	12	1	25

FOOD: (See Beverages & Fast Food Restaurants listed separately)	Serving Size	Cal- ories	Fat (g)	Carb (g)	Fi- ber (g)	Pro- tein (g)
Beef Jerky, ¾ oz	1	80	5	2	Tr	7
Beef Meals – see Hamburger	…	…	.	.	.	.
Helper for ground beef meals	…	…	.	.	.	.
Beef Oriental, Lean Cuisine	1 meal	270	8	30	3	20
Beef Patties, Banquet entrée	1 meal	180	14	7	Tr	8
Beef Peppercorn, Lean Cuisine	1 meal	260	7	32	1	16
Beef Portabello, Lean Cuisine	1 meal	220	7	24	1	14
Beef Romanoff	1 cup	290	11	28	2	20
Beef Stew w/ Vegetables	1 cup	215	12	16	4	11
Beef Stroganoff, Stouffers entrée	1 meal	390	20	30	1	23
Beef Teriyaki w/ vegetables	1 cup	250	10	22	3	18
Beef Tips, Healthy Choice entrée	1 meal	260	6	32	1	20
Beef w/ Broccoli, Hunan style	1 cup	250	8	30	3	18
Beef w/Vegetables, Szechuan	1 cup	270	8	30	3	20
Beet Greens, chopped, cooked	½ cup	20	Tr	4	2	2
Beets	…	…	.	.	.	.
Fresh, cooked, slices	½ cup	38	Tr	8	2	2
Fresh, cooked, whole beet, 2" dia	1 whole	22	Tr	5	1	1
Canned, drained, slices	½ cup	27	Tr	6	1	1
Canned, drained, whole beet	1 whole	12	Tr	2	Tr	1
Biscuit, plain or buttermilk	…	…	.	.	.	.
Prep from recipe, 2 ½" dia	1	210	10	27	1	4
Prep from recipe, 4" dia	1	360	16	45	2	7
Refrigerated dough, baked	…	…	.	.	.	.
regular 2 ½" dia	1	95	4	13	Tr	2
reduced fat, 2 ¼" dia	1	65	1	12	Tr	2
Biscuit w/ Bacon	1	360	4	27	1	9
Biscuit w/ Egg & Sausage	1	540	37	32	1	19
Biscuit w/ Ham	1	330	20	28	1	12
Biscuit w/ Sausage	1	460	33	28	1	12
Blackberries	…	…	.	.	.	.
Fresh	1 cup	75	1	18	8	1
Frozen, no sugar added, thawed	1 cup	80	1	19	8	1
Blueberries	…	…	.	.	.	.
Fresh	1 cup	80	1	20	4	1
Frozen, sugar sweetened, thawed	1 cup	185	Tr	50	5	1
Bologna (thin 1/8" slices)	…	…	.	.	.	.
Beef or Pork, regular	2 slices	180	16	2	0	7
Beef or Pork, lowfat	2 slices	110	9	2	0	6
Beef or Pork, fat free	2 slices	60	1	3	0	8

FOOD: (See Beverages & Fast Food Restaurants listed separately)	Serving Size	Cal-ories	Fat (g)	Carb (g)	Fi-ber (g)	Pro-tein (g)
Chicken or Turkey , regular	2 slices	160	14	2	0	7
Chicken or Turkey, lowfat	2 slices	100	8	2	0	6
Chicken or Turkey, fat free	2 slices	60	1	3	0	8
Bouillon - see Soup	...	...	.	.	.	.
Bratwurst, Boars Head	1 wurst	300	25	0	0	19
Braunschweiger, 2 avg slices	2 oz	205	18	2	Tr	8
BREAD	...	...	.	.	.	.
(avg ½" thick slice unless noted)	...	...	.	.	.	.
Banana bread, 1 ¼" slice	1 slice	195	6	33	1	3
Boston brown	1 slice	88	1	20	2	2
Bran'ola	1 slice	90	2	18	2	3
Bun, frankfurter, 1.4 oz, 5" long	1 bun	100	2	18	2	3
Bun, hamburger, 1.4 oz, 3 ½" dia	1 bun	100	2	18	2	3
Bun, Lg, 7" long or 4" dia round	1 bun	200	4	36	4	6
Carb Style, Pepperidge Farms	1 slice	60	2	8	3	5
Carrot bread	1 slice	200	9	28	2	3
Cinnamon raisin bread	1 slice	90	2	18	2	2
Cornbread, 3" x 2"	1 piece	185	6	29	1	4
Cracked wheat bread	1 slice	65	1	12	1	2
Croissant, butter flavor, 4"	1	230	12	26	2	5
Egg bread, ¾" slice	1 slice	115	2	19	1	4
English muffin, regular	1 whole	135	1	26	2	4
English muffin, cinnamon/raisin	1 whole	140	2	28	2	4
French bread	1 slice	70	1	13	1	2
Garlic bread, ¾" thick	1 slice	150	8	16	1	3
Italian bread	1 slice	65	1	12	1	2
Multigrain bread	1 slice	65	1	12	2	3
Oat/Oatmeal bread	1 slice	73	1	13	1	2
Pita bread, 4" pita	1 whole	77	Tr	16	1	3
Pita bread, 6 ½" pita	1 whole	165	1	33	1	5
Potato bread	1 slice	100	2	18	2	3
Pumpernickel bread	1 slice	80	1	15	2	3
Raisin bread	1 slice	100	1	19	2	3
Reduced calorie bread	1 slice	45	Tr	10	2	2
Roll, cinnamon, w/glaze, 3" dia	1 roll	200	7	33	1	4
Roll, hard or kaiser	1 roll	170	2	30	1	6
Roll, soft, avg size, 1.4 oz	1 roll	100	1	18	2	2
Rye bread	1 slice	75	1	14	2	3
Sourdough bread	1 slice	70	1	13	1	2
Submarine bread, 7" long	1	200	4	36	4	6
Vienna bread	1 slice	70	1	13	1	2

FOOD: (See Beverages & Fast Food Restaurants listed separately)	Serving Size	Cal- ories	Fat (g)	Carb (g)	Fi- ber (g)	Pro- tein (g)
Wheat bread	1 slice	65	1	12	1	2
White bread	1 slice	65	1	12	1	2
White or Wheat, light bread	1 slice	45	Tr	10	2	2
(also see Bagel & Biscuit)	...	...	.	.	.	.
Bread Crumbs	...	...	.	.	.	.
Dry, grated	1 cup	430	6	78	3	14
Dry, seasoned, grated	1 cup	440	3	84	5	17
Soft crumbs	1 cup	120	2	22	2	4
Bread Stick	...	...	.	.	.	.
Crunchy w/sesame seeds, 0.4 oz	1	40	1	7	1	1
Soft, pizza flavored, 1.5 oz	1	130	4	20	1	3
Bread Stuffing – see Stuffing or	...	...	.	.	.	.
Bread Crumbs	...	...	.	.	.	.
Breakfast Sandwich, bacon, egg,	...	...	.	.	.	.
& cheese on English muffin	1 avg	370	28	19	2	15
(also see Biscuit sandwiches)	...	...	.	.	.	.
Broccoli	...	...	.	.	.	.
Fresh, raw, flowerets	3	9	Tr	3	1	Tr
Fresh, raw, spear, 5" long	1	9	Tr	2	1	1
Fresh, raw, chopped or diced	1 cup	25	Tr	5	3	3
Fresh, cooked, spear, 5" long	1	10	Tr	2	1	1
Fresh, chopped, cooked	1 cup	44	1	8	5	5
Frozen, flowerets & cuts, cooked	1 cup	52	Tr	10	6	6
Prep w/ butter sauce	½ cup	75	5	6	3	2
Broccoli & Rice Casserole	¾ cup	240	12	26	5	5
Broccoli Au gratin	½ cup	100	4	10	3	5
Broth - see Soup	...	...	.	.	.	.
Brownie, 2" square	...	...	.	.	.	.
With frosting	1 square	190	8	27	1	2
Without frosting	1 square	140	6	20	1	2
Fat Free	1 square	90	Tr	22	1	1
Brussels Sprouts	...	...	.	.	.	.
Fresh, cooked	1 cup	61	1	14	4	4
Frozen, cooked	1 cup	65	1	13	6	6
Prep w/ butter	½ cup	75	3	8	3	3
Bugles (snacks)	...	...	.	.	.	.
Regular	1 ¼ cup	150	7	20	1	1
Baked	1 ¼ cup	130	4	23	1	2
Nacho	1 ¼ cup	160	9	18	1	2
Ranch	1 ¼ cup	160	9	18	1	2
Sour cream & onion	1 ¼ cup	160	9	20	1	2

FOOD: (See Beverages & Fast Food Restaurants listed separately)	Serving Size	Cal-ories	Fat (g)	Carb (g)	Fi-ber (g)	Pro-tein (g)
Bulgur	...	...	.	.	.	.
Cooked	1 cup	150	Tr	34	8	6
Uncooked	1 cup	480	2	106	26	17
Bun - see Bread	...	...	.	.	.	.
Burrito	...	...	.	.	.	.
Bean & cheese	1	275	15	25	2	10
Bean & green chili	1	270	9	35	3	10
Beans & rice	1	200	3	36	2	6
Beef & bean	1	300	17	26	2	11
Beef & cheese	1	300	18	26	2	10
Chicken	1	260	10	28	2	7
Butter (also see margarine)	...	...	.	.	.	.
Regular stick, 4 sticks/pound	1 stick	815	92	Tr	0	1
Regular, salted or unsalted	1 Tbsp	100	12	Tr	0	Tr
Regular, salted or unsalted	1 tsp	34	4	Tr	0	Tr
Apple Butter	1 Tbsp	30	0	7	Tr	Tr
Cabbage	...	...	.	.	.	.
Green, raw, shredded	1 cup	18	Tr	4	2	1
Green, chopped, cooked	1 cup	33	1	7	4	2
Chinese cabbage (bok choy)	...	...	.	.	.	.
shredded, raw	1 cup	10	Tr	2	2	1
shredded, cooked	1 cup	20	Tr	3	3	3
Red cabbage, raw, shredded	1 cup	19	Tr	4	1	1
Savoy cabbage, raw, shredded	1 cup	19	Tr	4	2	1
Cabbage, Stuffed w/ beef or pork	1 avg	100	3	9	2	6
CAKE	...	...	.	.	.	.
(average size slice of single layer	...	...	.	.	.	.
cake, 1/8 of 9", unless noted)	...	.	.	.	.	.
Angelfood cake, w/o frosting,	1 piece	125	Tr	28	Tr	3
Boston Cream Cake	1 piece	230	8	39	1	2
Carrot Cake, cream cheese icing	1 piece	485	29	52	2	5
Cheesecake, 1/6 of 17 oz cake	1 piece	260	18	20	Tr	5
Cheesecake w/chocolate, Lg slice	1 piece	580	41	44	1	9
Chocolate Cake	...	...	.	.	.	.
w/frosting	1 piece	390	13	70	2	5
w/o frosting	1 piece	290	11	44	2	5
Coffee Crumb Cake, 2.2 oz	1 piece	265	15	29	1	4
Cupcake – see Cupcakes	...	...	.	.	.	.
Devil's Food cake w/frosting	1 piece	395	13	71	2	5
Fat Free Cake,	...	...	.	.	.	.
Chocolate or Vanilla	...	...	.	.	.	.

FOOD: (See Beverages & Fast Food Restaurants listed separately)	Serving Size	Cal- ories	Fat (g)	Carb (g)	Fi- ber (g)	Pro- tein (g)
w/o frosting	1 piece	80	Tr	17	Tr	2
w/sugar free glaze	1 piece	85	Tr	18	Tr	2
Fruitcake, small slice	1 piece	160	5	27	2	1
Gingerbread	1 piece	265	12	36	1	3
Hummingbird	1 piece	595	30	72	1	5
Marble cake, w/o frosting	1 piece	255	12	34	1	3
Pineapple Upside Down Cake	1 piece	365	14	58	1	4
Pound Cake w/o glaze	1 piece	220	11	29	Tr	3
Shortcake, 3" dia	1 piece	225	9	32	1	4
Sponge Cake	1 piece	180	3	35	Tr	5
White Cake,	…	…	.	.	.	.
w/frosting	1 piece	395	12	71	1	5
w/o frosting	1 piece	265	9	42	1	4
Yellow Cake,	…	…	.	.	.	.
w/frosting	1 piece	390	12	70	1	5
w/o frosting	1 piece	260	9	42	1	4
CANDY	…	…	.	.	.	.
Atomic FireBall, ¾" dia	1	24	0	6	0	0
Almond Joy, 1.7 oz bar	1 bar	240	13	29	2	2
Baby Ruth, 2.1 oz bar	1 bar	290	13	39	1	5
Bit-O-Honey, 2.1 oz	1 bar	185	4	39	Tr	1
BreathSavers, sugar free	1	5	0	2	0	0
Butterfinger, 2.1 oz bar	1 bar	280	8	41	2	8
Candy Cane, 0.5 oz	1 cane	55	0	14	0	0
Candy Corn	¼ cup	180	1	45	0	0
Caramel	…	…	.	.	.	.
regular caramel, 0.3 oz	1 piece	35	1	7	Tr	Tr
regular caramel, 2.5 oz	2.5 oz	270	6	55	1	3
chocolate caramel, 0.3 oz	1 piece	25	Tr	6	Tr	Tr
Carob	1 oz	155	9	16	1	2
Charms Blow Pop	1	60	0	14	0	0
Chewing Gum-see Chewing Gum	…	…	.	.	.	.
Chocolate Bars	…	…	.	.	.	.
Hershey's Chocolate bar,	…	…	.	.	.	.
plain, 1.5 oz bar	1 bar	230	13	25	1	3
Hershey's Nugget, 10g	1 bar	52	3	6	Tr	1
Hershey's Snack Size, 17g	1 bar	90	5	10	Tr	1
with almonds, 1.45 oz	1 bar	220	14	22	3	4
with crispy rice, 1.55 oz	1 bar	230	12	29	1	3
with peanuts, 1.75 oz	1 bar	265	17	25	2	5
(see 'Chocolate for Baking'	…	…	.	.	.	.

FOOD: (See Beverages & Fast Food Restaurants listed separately)	Serving Size	Cal- ories	Fat (g)	Carb (g)	Fi- ber (g)	Pro- tein (g)
listed separately)	...	...	.	.	.	.
Chocolate Coated Peanuts	10	205	13	20	2	5
Chocolate Coated Raisins	10	40	1	7	2	Tr
Chocolate Kiss, Hershey's	4	102	6	11	Tr	1
Fifth Avenue bar, 2 oz	1 bar	195	8	26	1	4
Fruit Leather Bar	1 oz	95	2	22	1	Tr
Fruit Leather, small roll	1 roll	50	Tr	12	1	Tr
Fudge, chocolate, 0.6 oz piece	1 piece	65	1	13	1	Tr
Goobers, 1.4 oz	1	200	13	6	0	5
Gumdrops ¾" dia	5	64	0	16	0	0
Gummy Bears	10	85	0	22	0	0
Gummy Worms	10	285	0	73	0	0
Hard Candy, regular, 1" dia	...	...	.	.	.	.
Butterscotch or Coffee flavor	2	42	0	10	0	0
Cinnamon, Fruit, or Mint flavor	2	40	0	10	0	0
Hard Candy, sugar free	...	...	.	.	.	.
Baskin Robbins, sugarfree	...	...	.	.	.	.
Fruit or Chocolate Mint	2	20	1	7	0	0
Brachs, sugar free Cinnamon	3	35	0	17	0	0
Life Savers, sugar free	4	30	0	14	0	0
Sweet 'N Low Fruit Flavors	5	30	0	14	0	0
Sweet 'N Low Butterscotch	5	30	0	15	0	0
Sweet 'N Low Coffee	5	30	0	14	0	0
Jawbreaker, regular size, ¾" dia	1	24	0	6	0	0
Jawbreaker, large size, 1" dia	1	40	0	9	0	0
Jelly Beans, regular size	10	100	Tr	25	0	0
Jelly Beans, small pieces	10	40	Tr	10	0	0
Candy (Continued)	...	...	.	.	.	.
Kit Kat bar, 1.5 oz	1 bar	215	11	27	Tr	3
Krackel bar, 1.5 oz	1 bar	220	12	25	1	3
Licorice, 1.4 oz pkg	1.4 oz	135	1	31	0	1
LifeSavers	2	20	0	5	0	0
Lollipop, Charms Blow Pop, 15g	1	60	0	14	0	0
Lollipop, large, 14 g	1	50	0	12	0	0
Lollipop, small, Dum Dum, 5 g	1	24	0	6	0	0
M&M candy, plain	10	34	1	5	Tr	Tr
M&M candy, w/ nuts	10	103	5	12	1	2
Mars Almond bar, 1.75 oz	1 bar	235	12	31	2	4
Marshmallow, avg size	1	23	0	6	0	0
Milky Way, regular size, 2.15 oz	1 bar	258	10	44	1	3
Milky Way, small, fun size	1 bar	76	3	13	Tr	1

FOOD: (See Beverages & Fast Food Restaurants listed separately)	Serving Size	Cal- ories	Fat (g)	Carb (g)	Fi- ber (g)	Pro- tein (g)
Mints, pastel, ½" square	10	75	0	18	0	0
Mounds, 1.9 oz bar	1 bar	255	13	31	2	2
Mr. Goodbar, 1.75 oz	1 bar	265	17	25	2	5
Oh Henry, 2 oz bar	1 bar	245	10	37	1	6
Nestle Crunch bar, 1.55 oz	1 bar	230	12	29	1	3
Peanut Brittle	1 oz	130	5	20	1	2
Peppermint Pattie, 1.5 oz	1 pattie	165	3	34	1	1
Raisinets, 1.6 oz pkg	1 pkg	185	7	32	6	2
Reese's Peanut Butter Cups	...	...	.	.	.	.
regular size cups	2 cups	245	14	25	1	5
miniature size cups	2 cups	42	2	4	Tr	1
Reese's Pieces, 1.6 oz pkg	1 pkg	225	9	28	1	6
Reese Sticks, 0.6 oz bar	1 bar	90	1	9	Tr	2
Rolo caramels	9 piece	220	11	28	1	3
Skittles, 2.3 oz pkg	1 pkg	265	3	59	Tr	0
Skor toffee bar, 1.4 oz	1 bar	220	2	23	Tr	13
Snickers bar, regular size, 2 oz	1 bar	275	14	34	1	5
Snickers bar, small fun size	1 bar	72	4	9	Tr	1
Special Dark, miniature bar	1 bar	46	3	5	Tr	Tr
Starburst Fruit Chews, 2 oz pkg	1 pkg	235	5	50	0	Tr
Starlight Mints, 1" dia	3	56	0	14	0	0
Sucker – see Lollipop	...	...	.	.	.	.
Three Musketeers, 2.1 oz bar	1 bar	250	8	46	Tr	2
Toffee, 1.4 oz bar	1 bar	220	13	23	1	2
Tootsie Roll, 1 oz	1 oz	110	6	15	Tr	1
Twizzlers, Cherry, 2.5 oz pkg	1 pkg	135	1	31	0	1
Cannelloni, Cheese	...	...	.	.	.	.
Lean Cuisine entrée	1 meal	250	6	30	2	16
Cantaloupe	...	...	.	.	.	.
Fresh, medium size, 5" dia	½	98	Tr	22	2	3
Fresh, wedge 1/8 melon	1 wedge	25	Tr	6	1	1
Fresh, cubed	1 cup	55	Tr	13	1	1
Carambola (starfruit)	...	...	.	.	.	.
Fresh, 3 ½", whole	1	30	Tr	7	3	Tr
Fresh, sliced	1 cup	36	Tr	8	3	1
Caramels – see candy	...	...	.	.	.	.
Carrot	...	...	.	.	.	.
Fresh, raw, whole, 7 ½" long	1	32	Tr	7	2	1
Fresh, raw, shredded	1 cup	47	Tr	11	3	1
Fresh, baby carrots	2	12	Tr	3	1	Tr
Fresh, cooked, slices	1 cup	65	Tr	14	5	2

FOOD: (See Beverages & Fast Food Restaurants listed separately)	Serving Size	Cal- ories	Fat (g)	Carb (g)	Fi- ber (g)	Pro- tein (g)
Frozen, cooked, slices	1 cup	69	Tr	15	5	2
Canned, drained, slices, cooked	1 cup	57	Tr	13	3	1
Glazed carrots	¾ cup	280	15	35	5	1
Cashew – see Nuts	...	...	.	.	.	.
Casserole, see specific listings	...	...	.	.	.	.
Catsup, regular	1 Tbsp	18	Tr	4	Tr	Tr
Restaurant size packet	1 pkt	10	Tr	3	Tr	Tr
Cauliflower	...	...	.	.	.	.
Fresh, raw, flowerets	3	9	Tr	3	1	Tr
Fresh, raw, chopped or diced	1 cup	25	Tr	5	3	2
Fresh, flowerets, cooked	3	12	Tr	2	1	1
Fresh, chopped, cooked	1 cup	30	Tr	5	3	2
Frozen, cuts, cooked	1 cup	35	Tr	7	5	3
Prep w/ butter	¾ cup	100	8	6	2	2
Prep w/ cheese sauce	¾ cup	110	8	6	2	4
Cavatelli	1 cup	400	2	77	1	14
Caviar – see Fish	...	...	.	.	.	.
Cayenne, dried spice	¼ tsp	1	0	Tr	Tr	Tr
Caesar Salad	4 oz	200	17	7	2	7
Celery	...	...	.	.	.	.
Fresh, raw, stalk, 7 ½" long	1 stalk	6	Tr	1	Tr	Tr
Fresh, raw, diced	1 cup	19	Tr	4	2	1
Cooked, stalk 7 ½" long	1 stalk	6	Tr	1	Tr	Tr
Cooked, diced pieces	1 cup	27	Tr	6	2	1
Celery Seed	1 tsp	8	1	1	Tr	Tr
CEREAL	...	...	.	.	.	.
All-Bran	½ cup	80	1	23	10	4
Apple Jacks	1 cup	116	Tr	27	1	1
Cap'n Crunch, regular	¾ cup	107	1	23	1	1
Crunchberries	¾ cup	104	1	22	1	1
Peanut Butter Crunchy	¾ cup	112	2	22	1	2
Cheerios Cereal, regular	1 cup	110	2	23	3	3
Apple Cinnamon Cheerios	¾ cup	118	2	25	2	2
Chex Cereal, Corn	1 cup	113	Tr	26	1	2
Honey Nut	¾ cup	117	1	26	Tr	2
Multi Bran	1 cup	170	1	39	5	4
Rice	1¼ cup	117	Tr	27	Tr	2
Wheat	1 cup	104	1	24	3	3
Cinnamon Toast Crunch	¾ cup	124	3	24	2	2
Cocoa Krispies	¾ cup	120	1	27	Tr	2
Cocoa Puffs	1 cup	120	1	27	Tr	1

FOOD: (See Beverages & Fast Food Restaurants listed separately)	Serving Size	Cal-ories	Fat (g)	Carb (g)	Fi-ber (g)	Pro-tein (g)
Corn Flakes	1 cup	105	Tr	24	1	2
Corn Pops	1 cup	118	Tr	28	Tr	1
Cream of Wheat, as prep	1 cup	130	Tr	27	1	4
Crispix	1 cup	108	Tr	25	1	2
Fruit Loops	1 cup	117	1	26	1	1
Frosted Flakes	1 cup	120	Tr	28	1	1
Frosted Mini Wheats	...	...	.	.	.	.
regular size	1 cup	175	1	42	6	5
bite size	1 cup	190	1	45	6	5
Cereal (Continued)	...	...	.	.	.	.
Golden Grahams	¾ cup	116	1	26	1	2
Granola Cereal, Nature Valley	¾ cup	250	10	36	4	6
Honey Nut Cheerios	1 cup	115	1	24	2	3
Kix Cereal, regular	1¼ cup	114	1	26	1	2
Kix Berry Berry	¾ cup	120	1	26	Tr	1
Life Cereal, regular	¾ cup	120	1	25	2	3
Life Cinnamon Cereal	1 cup	190	2	40	3	4
Lucky Charms	1 cup	116	1	25	1	2
Malt O Meal, as prep	1 cup	122	Tr	26	1	4
Oat Cereal, Cheerios type	1 cup	110	2	23	3	3
Oatmeal, warm - see Oatmeal	...	...	.	.	.	.
Peanut Butter Puffed Cereal	¾ cup	130	3	23	Tr	3
Product 19	1 cup	110	Tr	25	1	3
Puffed Rice Cereal	1 cup	56	Tr	13	Tr	1
Puffed Wheat Cereal	1 cup	44	Tr	10	1	2
Raisin Bran Cereal	1 cup	180	1	45	7	1
Raisin Nut Bran	1 cup	210	4	41	5	5
Rice Crispies	1 ¼ cup	124	Tr	29	Tr	2
Shredded Wheat cereal,	...	...	.	.	.	.
large frosted biscuits	2 pc	155	1	38	5	5
Smacks Cereal	¾ cup	105	Tr	24	1	2
Special K	1 cup	115	Tr	22	1	6
Total	¾ cup	105	1	24	3	3
Trix Cereal	1 cup	122	2	26	1	1
Wheat Bran Flakes	¾ cup	95	1	23	5	3
Wheaties	1 cup	110	1	24	2	3
Cereal Bar	...	...	.	.	.	.
Plain	1 bar	135	2	28	1	2
Fruit filled	1 bar	145	2	29	1	2
Chalupa	...	...	.	.	.	.
Beef	1	380	23	29	2	14

FOOD: (See Beverages & Fast Food Restaurants listed separately)	Serving Size	Cal- ories	Fat (g)	Carb (g)	Fi- ber (g)	Pro- tein (g)
Chicken	1	360	20	28	2	17
Nacho cheese & beef	1	370	22	30	2	13
Nacho cheese & chicken	1	350	19	29	2	16
Nacho cheese & steak	1	350	19	28	2	16
CHEESE	...	...	.	.	.	.
American, pasteurized cheese	...	...	.	.	.	.
regular	1 oz	105	9	1	0	6
fat free	1 slice	25	0	3	0	4
Blue cheese	1 oz	100	8	1	0	6
Camembert 1.3 oz	1 wedge	114	9	Tr	0	8
Cheddar cheese	...	...	.	.	.	.
regular, 1 ounce slice	1 slice	115	9	Tr	0	7
1 inch cube	1 slice	68	6	Tr	0	4
shredded	1 cup	455	37	1	0	28
lowfat	1 oz	50	2	1	0	7
fat free	1 slice	25	0	3	0	4
Cheese food, pasteurized	1 oz	93	7	2	0	6
Cheese spread, pasteurized	1 oz	82	6	2	0	5
Colby cheese	1 oz	112	9	1	0	7
Cottage cheese	...	...	.	.	.	.
regular, creamed, 4% fat	...	...	.	.	.	.
large curd	1 cup	233	10	6	0	28
small curd	1 cup	217	9	6	0	26
with fruit	1 cup	279	8	30	0	22
lowfat, 2% fat	1 cup	203	4	8	0	31
lowfat, 1% fat	1 cup	164	2	6	0	28
fat free	1 cup	160	0	10	0	30
dry curd, uncreamed, 0.5% fat	1 cup	123	1	3	0	25
Cream cheese	...	...	.	.	.	.
regular cream	1 oz	100	10	1	0	2
regular cream	1 Tbsp	50	5	Tr	0	1
lowfat/light	1 Tbsp	35	3	1	0	2
fat free	1 Tbsp	15	0	1	0	2
Feta cheese	1 oz	75	6	1	0	4
Fontina cheese	1 oz	110	9	1	0	7
Goat cheese, soft	1 oz	75	6	1	0	4
Jalapeno jack cheese, processed	1 oz	90	8	1	0	5
Cheese (Continued)	...	...	.	.	.	.
Monterey jack cheese, processed	1 oz	105	9	Tr	0	7
Mozzarella cheese	...	...	.	.	.	.
regular, 1 ounce slice	1 slice	80	5	1	0	8

FOOD: (See Beverages & Fast Food Restaurants listed separately)	Serving Size	Cal-ories	Fat (g)	Carb (g)	Fi-ber (g)	Pro-tein (g)
shredded, 2 oz	½ cup	160	10	2	0	16
fat free	1 slice	25	0	3	0	4
Muenster cheese	…	…	.	.	.	.
sliced	1 oz	105	9	Tr	0	7
Neufchatel cheese	1 oz	75	7	1	0	3
Parmesan cheese	…	…	.	.	.	.
grated	1 cup	455	30	4	0	42
grated	1 Tbsp	25	2	Tr	0	2
Provolone cheese	1 oz	100	8	1	0	7
Ricotta cheese	…	…	.	.	.	.
regular	1 cup	430	32	7	0	28
part skim	1 cup	340	19	13	0	28
fat free	1 cup	240	0	20	0	40
Romano cheese, grated	1 oz	110	8	1	0	9
Roquefort, sheep's milk	1 oz	105	9	1	0	6
Swiss cheese	…	…	.	.	.	.
regular, 1 ounce slice	1 slice	105	8	1	0	8
fat free	1 slice	25	0	3	0	4
Cheese Puffs (about 25)	1 oz	160	10	15	Tr	2
Cheese Puffs Balls (2 ½ cups)	1 oz	160	10	15	Tr	2
Cheese Spread	…	…	.	.	.	.
Cheez Whiz	2 Tbsp	90	7	2	0	5
Velveeta	2 Tbsp	80	6	3	0	5
Cheetos (snacks)	…	…	.	.	.	.
Curls (about 15)	1 oz	150	10	15	Tr	2
Puffs (about 25)	1 oz	160	10	15	Tr	2
Cherries	…	…	.	.	.	.
Fresh, sweet	10	50	1	11	2	1
Sour, canned, water pack	1 cup	90	Tr	22	3	2
Cherry Pie Filling, canned	3 oz	80	Tr	20	Tr	Tr
Chestnut – see Nuts	…	…	.	.	.	.
Chewing Gum	…	…	.	.	.	.
Stick Gum, 2 ¾" long, all flavors	…	…	.	.	.	.
Wrigley's, regular	1 stick	10	0	2	0	0
Wrigley's Extra, sugarfree	1 stick	5	0	2	0	0
Carefree, sugarfree	1 stick	5	0	2	0	0
Bubble Yum, all regular flavors	1	25	0	6	0	0
Dentyne Ice, all flavors	2	5	0	2	0	0
Gum Balls, small, ½" dia balls	5	40	0	10	0	0
Gum Balls, Lg, 1 ¼" dia balls	1	32	0	8	0	0
Grapermelon, Wrigley's, ¾"	2	10	0	2	0	0

FOOD: (See Beverages & Fast Food Restaurants listed separately)	Serving Size	Cal-ories	Fat (g)	Carb (g)	Fi-ber (g)	Pro-tein (g)
Strappleberry, Wrigley's , ¾"	2	10	0	2	0	0
Trident, all flavors, 1" sticks	1 stick	5	0	1	0	0
Chex Mix, 1 oz	2/3 cup	120	5	18	2	3
CHICKEN	...	...	.	.	.	.
Giblets, simmered, chopped	1 cup	230	7	1	0	37
Fried Chicken, batter dipped	...	...	.	.	.	.
½ Breast, about 5 oz meat	½ breast	365	18	13	Tr	35
Drumstick, avg size	1	195	11	6	Tr	16
Thigh, avg size	1	240	14	8	Tr	19
Wing, avg size	1	160	11	5	Tr	10
Strips, dark meat	3 oz	205	9	10	Tr	25
Strips, white meat	3 oz	175	5	7	Tr	25
Liver of chicken, simmered	1	31	1	Tr	0	5
Neck, simmered	1	32	1	0	0	4
Roasted or Broiled Chicken	...	...	.	.	.	.
½ Breast, about 3.5 oz meat	½ breast	165	4	0	0	32
Drumstick, avg size	1	75	2	0	0	12
Thigh, avg size	1	110	6	0	0	13
White meat w/ skin	3.5 oz	280	12	0	0	33
White meat, skinless	3.5 oz	170	4	0	0	33
Dark meat w/ skin	3.5 oz	320	21	0	0	22
Dark meat skinless	3.5 oz	190	10	0	0	22
Canned, boneless	5 oz	235	11	0	0	31
Stewed Chicken	...	...	.	.	.	.
Light & dark meat, diced	1 cup	330	17	0	0	43
Wings, Buffalo, hot	3	210	12	3	0	22
Wings, Buffalo, mild	4	200	12	0	0	23
(Other Chicken Products, see:	...	...	.	.	.	.
Bologna, Hot Dog, Salami,	...	...	.	.	.	.
Sausage & specific entrées)	...	...	.	.	.	.
Chicken a la King	1 cup	320	22	17	Tr	15
Chicken Alfredo	1 cup	300	10	35	Tr	18
Chicken & Broccoli Alfredo	1 ½ cup	300	6	38	1	25
Chicken Cacciatoré	...	...	.	.	.	.
Healthy Choice entrée	1 meal	250	3	36	1	21
Lean Cuisine entrée	1 meal	280	10	25	1	23
Chicken Cordon Blue	...	...	.	.	.	.
Le Menu entrée	1 meal	460	20	48	1	23
Chicken Dijon, Healthy Choice	1 meal	270	5	33	1	23
Chicken Francesca	...	...	.	.	.	.
Healthy Choice entrée	1 meal	330	6	46	1	23

FOOD: (See Beverages & Fast Food Restaurants listed separately)	Serving Size	Cal-ories	Fat (g)	Carb (g)	Fi-ber (g)	Pro-tein (g)
Chicken Kiev, Tyson entrée	1 meal	440	25	36	1	18
Chicken Marsala, Tyson entrée	1 meal	180	5	19	1	15
Chicken Nuggets	…	…	.	.	.	.
Banquet entrée	1 meal	410	21	38	1	18
Morton entrée	1 meal	320	17	30	1	13
Chicken Parmagiana	…	…	.	.	.	.
Banquet entrée	1 meal	290	15	27	1	14
Healthy Choice entrée	1 meal	300	4	47	1	20
Le Menu entrée	1 meal	395	19	30	1	26
Chicken Roll, light meat	2 oz	90	4	2	1	11
Chicken Teriyaki w/vegetables	1 cup	200	8	20	2	12
Chicken w/Sweet & Sour Sauce	1 cup	320	5	53	2	19
Chicken w/Vegetables	…	.	.	.	.	.
Lean Cuisine entrée	1 meal	250	5	33	2	18
Chickpeas, cooked	½ cup	140	2	25	6	7
Chili Powder	1 tsp	8	Tr	1	Tr	Tr
Chili w/Beans	1 cup	270	11	23	8	21
Con Carne w/Beans	1 cup	255	8	24	8	20
Chimichanga	…	…	.	.	.	.
Beans & cheese	1	300	17	25	1	9
Beef & cheese	1	425	20	43	1	20
Chicken & cheese	1	350	16	39	1	11
Chips – see Corn Chips, Potato	…	…	.	.	.	.
Chips & other specific listings	…	…	.	.	.	.
Chives, raw, chopped	1 Tbsp	1	Tr	Tr	Tr	Tr
Chocolate for Baking (Also see	…	…	.	.	.	.
'Candy' for other chocolates)	…	…	.	.	.	.
Chocolate Chips, milk, regular	1 cup	860	52	99	6	12
Chocolate Chips, semisweet	1 cup	805	50	106	10	7
Chocolate Chips, white	1 cup	915	55	101	0	10
Unsweetened for baking, solid	1 square	148	16	8	4	3
Unsweetened, liquid	1 oz	134	14	10	5	3
Chow Mein	…	…	.	.	.	.
Beef chow mein	1 ½ cup	170	6	12	2	14
Chicken chow mein	1 ½ cup	160	7	12	2	14
Cilantro, raw	1 tsp	Tr	Tr	Tr	Tr	Tr
Cinnamon	1 tsp	6	Tr	2	1	Tr
Cinnamon Sweet Roll	…	…	.	.	.	.
With glaze, 3" dia	1	200	7	33	1	4
With raisins & glaze, 3" dia	1	225	10	35	1	4

FOOD: (See Beverages & Fast Food Restaurants listed separately)	Serving Size	Cal-ories	Fat (g)	Carb (g)	Fi-ber (g)	Pro-tein (g)
With raisins & glaze, 4 ½" dia	1	510	15	85	2	8
Clam Chowder - see Soup	...	...	.	.	.	.
Clams – see Fish/Seafood	...	...	.	.	.	.
Cloves, ground	1 tsp	6	Tr	1	Tr	Tr
Cocoa, unsweetened powder	1 Tbsp	15	1	3	2	1
	1 cup	240	16	48	32	16
Coconut	...	...	.	.	.	.
Fresh piece, 2" x 2" x ½"	1 piece	160	15	7	4	1
Fresh, shredded, not packed	1 cup	285	27	12	7	3
Dried, sweetened, flaked	1 cup	465	33	44	4	3
Coleslaw	½ cup	62	2	10	1	1
Collards	...	...	.	.	.	.
Fresh, chopped, cooked	1 cup	49	1	9	5	4
Frozen, chopped, cooked	1 cup	61	1	12	5	5
Condiments, see Sauce, or see specific listing	...	...	.	.	.	.
COOKIES 2 ¼" dia unless noted	...	...	.	.	.	.
Animal Crackers, 1" dia	8	60	1	12	Tr	1
Butter Cookie	1	50	2	7	Tr	Tr
Chocolate Chip, regular	1	80	3	12	1	2
Chocolate Chip, reduced fat	1	70	1	12	1	2
Chocolate Chip, sugar free	1	70	6	10	1	1
Coconut cookie	1	75	3	11	1	1
Fig Newton	2	110	2	20	1	1
Molasses cookie	1	80	2	13	Tr	1
Oatmeal w/ raisins	1	75	2	12	1	1
Oatmeal, plain	1	70	2	11	1	1
Oatmeal, sugarfree	1	70	6	10	1	1
Peanut Butter, plain	1	80	2	10	Tr	1
Peanut Butter w/ nuts	1	90	3	11	Tr	2
Pecan Shortbread cookie	1	75	5	8	Tr	1
Sandwich cookie, w/ filling, 1 ½" dia, round,	...	...	.	.	.	.
chocolate w/ creme filling	1	50	2	7	Tr	Tr
sugar w/ peanut butter filling	1	60	2	8	Tr	1
vanilla w/ creme filling	1	50	2	7	Tr	Tr
Shortbread cookie, plain	1	45	2	6	Tr	Tr
Shortbread w/fudge stripes	1	65	3	9	Tr	Tr
Sugar Cookie, regular	1	65	3	8	Tr	1
Sugar Cookie, reduced fat	1	55	1	9	Tr	1
Wafer, creme filled,	...	...	.	.	.	.

FOOD: (See Beverages & Fast Food Restaurants listed separately)	Serving Size	Cal-ories	Fat (g)	Carb (g)	Fi-ber (g)	Pro-tein (g)
2 ½" x 1" rectangles,	...	...	.	.	.	.
chocolate, creme filling	3	140	7	18	1	1
sugarfree, w/ filling	3	100	8	14	Tr	1
vanilla, creme filling	3	130	6	19	Tr	1
Wafer, Vanilla, round, 1 ½" dia	4	75	3	10	Tr	1
Cooking Spray, nonstick	...	...	.	.	.	.
¼ second spray	1 spray	0	0	0	0	0
Corn	...	...	.	.	.	.
Sweet White, 5" cob, cooked	1 ear	83	1	19	2	3
Sweet Yellow, on 5" cob,	...	...	.	.	.	.
fresh, cooked, 5" cob	1 ear	83	1	19	2	3
frozen, cooked, 5" cob	1 ear	75	1	18	2	2
frozen, cooked, kernels	½ cup	65	Tr	16	2	2
canned, kernels, vacuum pack	½ cup	83	1	20	2	3
canned, cream style kernels	½ cup	92	1	23	2	2
Prep w/butter & herb sauce	¾ cup	180	4	30	2	5
Corn Cake, butter flavor	1	40	Tr	8	1	1
(also see Rice Cake)	...	...	.	.	.	.
Corn Chips	...	...	.	.	.	.
Regular	1 oz	160	10	15	1	2
Barbecue flavor	1 oz	170	10	17	1	2
Ranch flavor	1 oz	150	7	20	1	2
Reduced fat	1 oz	130	5	22	1	2
Tortilla type	1 oz	140	7	17	1	2
Doritos corn chips	12 chips	140	7	18	1	2
Doritos nacho cheese	12 chips	140	7	18	1	2
Doritos ranch	12 chips	140	7	18	1	2
Doritos spicy nacho	12 chips	135	6	18	1	2
Fritos corn chips, regular	28 chips	160	10	15	1	2
Fritos BBQ corn chips	28 chips	160	9	16	1	2
Fritos Chili cheese corn chips	28 chips	160	10	15	1	2
Tostitos corn chips, round	13 chips	150	6	19	1	2
Tostitos baked	13 chips	110	1	21	1	3
Tostitos nacho	6 chips	150	6	19	1	2
Tostitos restaurant style	7 chips	140	6	19	1	2
Corn Grits (hominy) – see Grits	...	...	.	.	.	.
Corn Syrup	1 Tbsp	56	0	15	0	0
Cornbread, 3" x 2"	1 piece	185	6	29	1	4
Corned Beef, canned	3 oz	215	13	0	0	23
Corned Beef Hash	1 cup	440	30	23	1	19
Cornish Hen, roasted	4 oz	200	14	0	0	19

FOOD: (See Beverages & Fast Food Restaurants listed separately)	Serving Size	Cal-ories	Fat (g)	Carb (g)	Fi-ber (g)	Pro-tein (g)
Cornmeal, yellow, dry form	...	...	.	.	.	.
Whole grain	1 cup	440	4	94	9	10
Self rising	1 cup	490	2	103	10	12
Cornstarch	1 Tbsp	30	Tr	7	Tr	Tr
Cottage cheese – see Cheese	...	...	.	.	.	.
Crabcake	1	150	4	12	Tr	9
Cracker Jacks	½ cup	120	2	23	2	2
CRACKERS	...	...	.	.	.	.
Butter flavor, round, 2" dia	5	80	4	10	Tr	1
Cheese crackers, 1" squares	10	50	3	6	Tr	1
Chicken in a Biskit	12	160	8	17	1	2
Club crackers	4	70	3	9	Tr	1
Club crackers, Keebler Club	4	50	2	6	Tr	Tr
Graham crackers, 2 ½" sq	3	90	2	16	Tr	1
Matzo, plain, 6" square	1	120	Tr	25	1	3
Melba toast, plain	4	80	1	15	Tr	2
Oat Thins	9	70	3	10	1	2
Oyster crackers	25	65	1	11	1	1
Ritz Bitz w/peanut butter	13	150	8	17	1	4
Ritz crackers, regular	5	80	4	10	Tr	1
Ritz crackers, reduced fat	5	70	2	11	Tr	1
Saltine crackers	4	50	1	9	Tr	1
Sandwich crackers, 1 ½" dia,	...	...	.	.	.	.
cheese filled	2	65	2	8	Tr	2
peanut butter filled	2	68	4	8	Tr	2
Snack crackers, round, 2" dia	5	80	4	10	Tr	1
Sociables	7	80	4	9	Tr	1
Town House crackers	5	80	4	9	Tr	1
Triscuit wafers	7	140	5	21	1	3
Vegetable crackers, thin squares	7	80	4	10	1	2
Wheat Thins	9	60	2	10	1	1
Wheatables	8	70	3	10	1	1
Whole wheat, thin squares	8	75	4	10	1	2
Zwieback	2	70	2	12	1	2
Cranberries	...	.	.	.	.	.
Fresh, raw, unsweetened	½ cup	23	Tr	5	2	Tr
Dried, sweetened	¼ cup	90	Tr	24	3	Tr
Cranberry Relish	¾ cup	330	5	70	2	1
Cranberry relish w/walnuts	¾ cup	365	6	75	3	3
Cranberry Sauce, sweet, canned	1 slice	85	Tr	22	1	Tr
Cream Cheese - see Cheese	...	...	.	.	.	.

FOOD: (See Beverages & Fast Food Restaurants listed separately)	Serving Size	Cal-ories	Fat (g)	Carb (g)	Fi-ber (g)	Pro-tein (g)
Cream of Tartar	1 tsp	8	0	2	Tr	0
Cream of Wheat Cereal, as prep	1 cup	130	Tr	27	1	4
Cream, Whipped Topping	.	.	.	.	.	.
Light	1 cup	700	75	7	0	5
Light	1 Tbsp	45	5	Tr	0	Tr
Heavy	1 cup	820	88	7	0	5
Heavy	1 Tbsp	50	6	Tr	0	Tr
Pressurized in can	1 Tbsp	8	1	Tr	0	Tr
Creamer-see Beverages, Creamer	...	...	.	.	.	.
Croissant, butter flavor, 4"	1	230	12	26	2	5
Croissant w/Egg, Bacon, Cheese	1	415	28	24	2	16
Croissant w/Sausage	1	440	32	29	2	13
Croutons, seasoned	½ cup	92	3	13	1	2
Cucumber	...	...	.	.	.	.
Fresh, peeled, whole, 8" long	1	35	Tr	7	2	2
Fresh, peeled, sliced	1 cup	14	Tr	3	1	1
Fresh, unpeeled, whole 8" long	1	40	Tr	8	2	2
Fresh, unpeeled, sliced	1 cup	14	Tr	3	1	1
Cucumber Salad, mayo dressing	¾ cup	120	10	9	2	2
Cupcake, w/frosting, avg size,	...	...	.	.	.	.
2 ¾" dia x 2 ¼" tall	...	...	.	.	.	.
Banana	1	190	6	32	1	1
Blueberry	1	185	6	30	1	1
Chocolate	1	195	6	32	1	2
Chocolate w/ crème filling	1	190	7	31	1	1
Coconut w/ crème filling	1	200	7	34	1	1
Strawberry	1	185	6	30	1	1
Vanilla	1	190	6	32	Tr	1
Curry Powder	1 tsp	7	Tr	1	Tr	Tr
Custard	½ cup	170	6	23	Tr	6
Dandelion Greens, cooked	1 cup	35	Tr	7	3	2
Danish Pastry	...	...	.	.	.	.
Cheese, 4" dia	1	265	15	26	1	6
Cinnamon & raisin, 4" dia	1	260	12	33	2	5
Fruit filled, 4" dia	1	260	12	34	1	4
Large, Cheese w/ fruit, 5" x 3"	1	425	18	55	2	8
Dates, pitted	...	...	.	.	.	.
Whole	5 dates	115	Tr	30	3	1
Chopped	1 cup	490	1	130	13	4
Dessert – see Ice Cream, Frozen	...	...	.	.	.	.

FOOD: (See Beverages & Fast Food Restaurants listed separately)	Serving Size	Cal-ories	Fat (g)	Carb (g)	Fi-ber (g)	Pro-tein (g)
Dessert, or specific listing	...	...	.	.	.	.
Dessert Filling - see specific listing	... ...	... ...	.	.	.	.
Dessert Topping – see Topping	...	...	.	.	.	.
Dill Weed, raw, sprigs	5	Tr	Tr	Tr	Tr	Tr
Dip	...	...	.	.	.	.
Avocado	1 Tbsp	30	2	2	Tr	1
Bacon	1 Tbsp	30	2	2	Tr	1
French Onion	1 Tbsp	25	2	1	Tr	Tr
Ranch	1 Tbsp	30	2	2	Tr	1
Sour Cream & Chives, regular	1 Tbsp	30	2	2	Tr	1
Sour Cream & Chives, light	1 Tbsp	15	Tr	2	Tr	1
Doughnut	...	...	.	.	.	.
Cake Doughnuts	...	...	.	.	.	.
Regular ring type, 3" dia	...	...	.	.	.	.
Plain	1	200	11	23	1	2
Powdered sugar	1	240	11	33	1	3
Chocolate frosting	1	270	13	36	1	3
Vanilla frosting & sprinkles	1	280	13	39	1	3
Holes or Munchkin type, small	...	...	.	.	.	.
Cinnamon coated	4	250	14	30	2	3
Plain	4	220	14	22	2	2
Powdered sugar	4	250	14	29	2	2
Cruller	...	...	.	.	.	.
Glazed & frosted w/chocolate	1	280	15	35	1	2
Yeast Doughnuts	...	...	.	...	.	.
Regular ring type, 3" dia	...	...	.	...	.	.
Glazed	1	200	12	22	1	2
Glazed & frosted w/vanilla	1	250	12	33	1	3
Glazed & frosted w/chocolate plus sprinkles	... 1	... 270	. 12	. 36	. 1	. 3
Holes or Munchkin type, small	...	...	.	.	.	.
Glazed	5	200	9	27	1	3
Sugar coated	6	220	12	26	1	4
Filled doughnuts	...	...	.	.	.	.
Vanilla iced, crème filled	1	360	19	41	2	5
Powdered & strawberry filled	1	260	16	26	1	3
Dressing – see Salad Dressing	...	...	.	.	.	.
Dried Fruit – see specific listings, and Trail Mix	... ...	... ...	.	.	.	.
Duck, roasted	...	.	.	.	.	.

FOOD: (See Beverages & Fast Food Restaurants listed separately)	Serving Size	Cal-ories	Fat (g)	Carb (g)	Fi-ber (g)	Pro-tein (g)
½ Duck, meat only	½ duck	445	25	0	0	52
Dumpling, w/fruit	1	290				
Éclair, 5" x 2"	1	260	16	24	1	6
EGG	...	...	.	.	.	.
Raw Eggs	...	...	.	.	.	.
1 medium whole egg	1	65	4	1	0	5
1 large whole egg	1	75	5	1	0	6
1 extra large whole egg	1	85	6	1	0	7
1 yolk only, large	1	60	5	Tr	0	3
1 white only, large	1	15	0	Tr	0	4
Prepared Eggs (1 Lg egg/svg)	...	...	.	.	.	.
deviled	1	120	10	1	0	7
hard boiled, whole	1	75	5	1	0	6
hard boiled, chopped	1 cup	210	14	2	0	17
omelet, plain, milk added	1	105	8	1	0	7
pan fried in margarine	1	92	7	1	0	6
poached	1	75	5	1	0	6
scrambled w/margarine & milk	1	100	7	1	0	7
Egg Substitute or imitation	¼ cup	35	1	Tr	0	6
Eggplant	...	...	.	.	.	.
Cubed, cooked	1 cup	28	Tr	7	3	1
Fried sticks	½ cup	240	12	28	3	4
Eggplant Parmagiana	½ cup	265	16	26	3	6
Eggroll	...	...	.	.	.	.
Chicken, Chun King entrée	1 meal	170	5	25	2	7
Chicken, La Choy entrée	1 meal	170	5	25	2	7
Pork, Chun King entrée	1 meal	170	6	23	2	6
Pork eggroll, 4" long, 1 avg	1	165	6	22	2	6
Shrimp, Chun King entrée	1 meal	150	4	24	2	6
Enchilada	...	...	.	.	.	.
Beef, Banquet entrée	1meal	380	12	54	1	15
Beef, Patio entrée	1 meal	350	10	52	1	12
Cheese, Banquet entrée	1 meal	340	6	56	1	15
Chicken, Banquet entrée	1 meal	360	10	54	1	15
Enchirito	...	...	.	.	.	.
Beef	1	370	19	33	2	18
Chicken	1	350	16	32	2	21
Steak	1	350	16	31	2	22
Endive, raw, chopped	1 cup	9	Tr	2	2	1
Energy Bar, low carb	...	...	.	.	.	.
Atkins Advantage Chocolate	1 bar	220	11	25	11	17

FOOD: (See Beverages & Fast Food Restaurants listed separately)	Serving Size	Cal-ories	Fat (g)	Carb (g)	Fi-ber (g)	Pro-tein (g)
Atkins Advantage S'mores	1 bar	220	10	26	11	17
English Muffin	...	...	.	.	.	.
Regular	1 whole	135	1	26	2	4
Cinnamon raisin	1 whole	140	2	28	2	4
English Muffin w/Egg, Cheese, & Canadian Bacon	... 1	... 290	. 13	. 27	. 2	. 17
Equal sweetener	1 pkt	0	0	Tr	0	0
Fajita, Chicken, Healthy Choice	1 meal	260	4	36	1	21
Fettuccini Alfredo, w/ beef	1 cup	310	13	26	2	20
Fig, fresh or dried, large	2	98	Tr	25	5	1
FISH / SEAFOOD	...	...	.	.	.	.
Abalone, fried	3 oz	160	6	9	1	17
Anchovy, canned in oil	5	42	2	0	0	6
Bass	...	...	.	.	.	.
black, baked	3 oz	260	16	11	0	16
striped, baked	3 oz	105	3	0	0	19
Bluefish, baked	3 oz	135	5	0	0	22
Catfish	...	...	.	.	.	.
baked or broiled	3 oz	130	5	0	0	20
breaded, fried	3 oz	195	8	17	1	13
Caviar, black or red	2 Tbsp	80	6	1	0	8
Clams	...	...	.	.	.	.
breaded, fried	¾ cup	450	26	39	Tr	13
canned, drained	3 oz	125	2	4	0	22
canned, drained	1 cup	235	3	8	0	41
raw	3 oz	63	1	2	0	11
raw	1 med	11	Tr	Tr	0	2
steamed	3 oz	125	2	4	0	22
Cod, baked or broiled	3 oz	90	1	0	0	20
Crab, Alaska king	...	...	.	.	.	.
steamed	3 oz	82	1	0	0	16
steamed	1 leg	130	2	0	0	26
Crab, blue	...	...	.	.	.	.
steamed	3 oz	88	2	0	0	17
canned	1 cup	135	2	0	0	28
Crab, imitation crab meat	3 oz	88	1	9	0	10
Crab cake, w/egg, fried	1 cake	95	5	1	0	12
Fish fillet, breaded, fried	3 oz	190	9	17	1	10
Fish stick, breaded, fried, 3" x 1"	2 sticks	76	3	7	Tr	4
Flounder	...	...	.	.	.	.
baked or broiled	3 oz	100	1	0	0	21

FOOD: (See Beverages & Fast Food Restaurants listed separately)	Serving Size	Cal- ories	Fat (g)	Carb (g)	Fi- ber (g)	Pro- tein (g)
breaded, fried fillet	3 oz	190	8	17	1	13
Grouper, baked or broiled	3 oz	100	1	0	0	21
Haddock	...	...	.	.	.	.
baked or broiled	3 oz	95	1	0	0	21
breaded, fried fillet	3 oz	195	8	17	1	13
Halibut	...	...	.	.	.	.
baked or broiled	3 oz	120	2	0	0	23
breaded, fried fillet	3 oz	210	9	17	1	14
Herring, pickled	3 oz	225	15	8	0	12
Lobster, steamed	3 oz	85	1	1	0	17
Lobster, imitation meat	3 oz	90	1	9	0	10
Mackerel	...	...	.	.	.	.
baked or broiled	3 oz	225	15	0	0	20
mackerel, jack, canned	1 cup	295	12	0	0	44
Monkfish, baked or broiled	3 oz	130	4	0	0	21
Mussels, steamed	3 oz	145	4	6	0	20
Orange roughy, baked or broiled	3 oz	75	1	0	0	16
Oyster	...	...	.	.	.	.
raw meat	1 cup	170	6	10	0	17
raw meat	6 med	55	2	3	0	6
breaded, fried	3 oz	165	11	10	1	7
Fish / Seafood (Continued)	...	...	.	.	.	.
Perch, baked or broiled	3 oz	105	2	0	0	20
Pike, baked or broiled	3 oz	95	1	0	0	21
Pollock, baked or broiled	3 oz	95	1	0	0	20
Pompano, baked or broiled	3 oz	180	10	0	0	20
Rockfish, baked or broiled	3 oz	105	2	0	0	20
Salmon	...	...	.	.	.	.
baked or broiled	3 oz	185	9	0	0	23
canned, pink	3 oz	118	5	0	0	17
smoked, chinook	3 oz	100	4	0	0	16
Sardine, canned in oil, drained	3 oz	175	10	0	0	21
Scallop	...	...	.	.	.	.
breaded, fried	6 large	200	10	9	Tr	17
steamed	3 oz	95	1	3	0	20
Shark	...	...	.	.	.	.
Pacific shark, baked	3 oz	130	8	0	0	15
thrasher, baked	3 oz	85	1	0	0	18
Shrimp	...	...	.	.	.	.
breaded, fried	2 large	110	6	5	Tr	10
breaded, fried	3 oz	205	10	10	Tr	18

FOOD: (See Beverages & Fast Food Restaurants listed separately)	Serving Size	Cal-ories	Fat (g)	Carb (g)	Fi-ber (g)	Pro-tein (g)
canned, drained	3 oz	100	2	1	0	20
Snapper, baked or broiled	3 oz	110	2	0	0	22
Sole	...	...	.	.	.	.
baked or broiled	3 oz	100	1	0	0	21
breaded, fried fillet	3 oz	190	8	17	1	13
Squid, fried	3 oz	150	6	7	0	15
Swordfish	...	...	.	.	.	.
baked	3 oz	130	4	0	0	22
broiled	4 oz	170	5	0	0	28
Trout, baked or broiled	3 oz	145	6	0	0	21
Tuna	...	...	.	.	.	.
baked or broiled	3 oz	120	1	0	0	25
canned in oil, drained	3 oz	170	7	0	0	25
canned in water, chunk light	3 oz	100	1	0	0	22
canned in water, solid white	3 oz	110	3	0	0	20
tuna salad, oil packed, w/mayo	½ cup	190	10	9	0	16
tuna salad, water packed, w/	...	...	.	.	.	.
light mayo type dressing	½ cup	130	5	6	0	15
Whiting, baked or broiled	3 oz	100	1	0	0	21
Fish & Chips, Swanson entrée	1 meal	495	20	60	2	20
Fish & Macaroni w/cheese	...	...	.	.	.	.
Stouffers entrée	1 meal	460	20	47	2	22
Fish Baked w/Lemon Pepper	...	...	.	.	.	.
Healthy Choice entrée	1 meal	290	5	47	1	14
Fish Florentine, Lean Cuisine	1 meal	240	9	13	Tr	27
Fish Sandwich, 3 oz fried fish	...	...	.	.	.	.
fillet with tarter sauce & cheese	1 avg	530	29	48	Tr	22
Flank Steak – see Beef	...	...	.	.	.	.
Flour, unsifted	...	...	.	.	.	.
All purpose flour, white	1 cup	455	1	95	3	13
Bread flour	1 cup	495	2	99	3	16
Buckwheat flour, whole groat	1 cup	400	4	85	12	15
Cake or pastry flour	1 cup	495	1	107	2	11
Carob flour	1 cup	230	1	92	41	5
Self-rising flour, white	1 cup	443	1	93	3	12
Whole wheat flour	1 cup	407	2	87	15	16
Frankfurter – see Hot Dog	...	...	.	.	.	.
Freezer Pop – see Frozen Dessert	...	...	.	.	.	.
French Fries	...	...	.	.	.	.
Frozen, heated,	...	...	.	.	.	.
thin, shoestring strips, 3 oz	20 fries	130	4	22	2	2

FOOD: (See Beverages & Fast Food Restaurants listed separately)	Serving Size	Cal- ories	Fat (g)	Carb (g)	Fi- ber (g)	Pro- tein (g)
thick or crinkle cuts, 4.5 oz	20 fries	195	6	33	3	3
Restaurant type, regular fries	1 med	350	15	48	5	5
Curly Cheddar Fries	1 med	460	24	54	5	6
Curly Fries	1 med	400	20	40	5	5
French Toast	2 slices	250	8	38	1	8
Fried Chicken – see Chicken	...	...	.	.	.	.
Fried Rice – see Rice	...	...	.	.	.	.
Frijoles	1 cup	225	8	29	2	11
Frosting	...	...	.	.	.	.
Chocolate	1 Tbsp	75	3	12	Tr	Tr
Vanilla	1 Tbsp	80	3	13	Tr	Tr
Frozen Dessert	...	...	.	.	.	.
(also see Ice Cream)	...	...	.	.	.	.
Freezer Pop – (long tubes)_	...	...	.	.	.	.
Regular, fruit flavored, 1.5 oz	1	25	0	6	0	0
Sugar free, fruit flavored, 1.5 oz	2	4	0	1	0	0
Frozen chocolate log cake	1 slice	280	9	43	1	5
Frozen chocolate round cake	1 slice	340	12	53	1	7
Fruit & Juice Bar, 2.5 oz	1	65	Tr	16	0	1
Fudge Bar, 1.75 oz	1	65	Tr	13	Tr	4
Ice Pop Bar, 2 oz	1	45	0	11	0	0
Italian Ices	½ cup	65	Tr	16	0	Tr
Popsicle, 4 oz	1	90	0	22	0	0
Vanilla Sandwich bar	1	220	9	31	1	4
Fruit (see specific listings)	...	...	.	.	.	.
Mixed, canned, w/light syrup	1 cup	150	Tr	39	2	2
Mixed, frozen, sweetened	1 cup	245	Tr	61	5	4
Fruit Cocktail	...	...	.	.	.	.
Canned in heavy syrup	1 cup	180	Tr	47	3	1
Canned in juice	1 cup	110	Tr	28	2	1
Fruit Salad, mixed diced fruits	¾ cup	70	1	9	3	1
Fudge	...	...	.	.	.	.
Chocolate fudge, plain	1 oz	110	2	24	Tr	1
Chocolate fudge w/ nuts	1 oz	125	4	21	Tr	2
Vanilla fudge, plain	1 oz	105	1	23	Tr	1
Vanilla fudge, w/nuts	1 oz	120	4	22	Tr	1
Funyuns (snacks)	13	140	7	18	1	2
Garlic, raw	1 clove	4	Tr	1	Tr	Tr
Garlic Powder or Salt	1 tsp	8	Tr	2	Tr	Tr
Gelatin (Jello)	...	...	.	.	.	.

FOOD: (See Beverages & Fast Food Restaurants listed separately)	Serving Size	Cal- ories	Fat (g)	Carb (g)	Fi- ber (g)	Pro- tein (g)
Banana, regular	½ cup	80	0	19	0	2
Banana, sugar free	½ cup	10	0	1	0	1
Cherry, regular	½ cup	75	0	18	0	2
Cherry, sugar free	½ cup	10	0	1	0	1
Orange, regular	½ cup	75	0	18	0	2
Orange, sugar free	½ cup	10	0	1	0	1
Raspberry, regular	½ cup	75	0	18	0	2
Raspberry, sugar free	½ cup	10	0	1	0	1
Strawberry , regular	½ cup	75	0	18	0	2
Strawberry, sugar free	½ cup	10	0	1	0	1
Gordita	...	...	.	.	.	.
Beef & cheese	1	310	15	30	2	13
Chicken & cheese	1	290	13	29	2	15
Steak & cheese	1	290	13	28	2	16
Granola Bar	...	...	.	.	.	.
Low fat, fruit variety	1 bar	90	1	19	2	3
Plain granola bar	1 bar	135	6	18	2	3
Chocolate chip	1 bar	150	6	22	1	3
Chocolate chip & peanuts	1 bar	160	10	18	2	4
Coconut	1 bar	140	6	20	1	3
Raisin	1 bar	140	6	20	1	3
Grapefruit, pink, red, or white	...	...	.	.	.	.
fresh, 3 ¾" dia	1	80	Tr	18	3	2
canned, in juice	1 cup	115	Tr	28	2	1
canned, in light syrup	1 cup	150	Tr	39	1	1
Grapes, seeded	...	...	.	.	.	.
Fresh, medium size, all types	10	35	Tr	9	1	Tr
Fresh, small or medium size	1 cup	115	1	28	2	1
Gravy	...	...	.	.	.	.
Beef	¼ cup	40	2	4	Tr	2
Chicken	¼ cup	32	1	3	Tr	2
Country Sausage	¼ cup	60	4	4	Tr	2
Mushroom	¼ cup	30	2	3	Tr	1
Pork	¼ cup	38	2	3	Tr	2
Turkey	¼ cup	31	1	3	Tr	2
Grits, corn (hominy), as prep	1 cup	145	Tr	31	1	3
Ground Beef – see Beef	...	...	.	.	.	.
Guava, raw, med size	1	45	Tr	11	2	1
Gum – see Chewing Gum	...	...	.	.	.	.
HAM (also see Pork)	...	...	.	.	.	.
Canned, regular, roasted	3 oz	155	9	2	0	15

FOOD: (See Beverages & Fast Food Restaurants listed separately)	Serving Size	Cal- ories	Fat (g)	Carb (g)	Fi- ber (g)	Pro- tein (g)
lean, roasted	3 oz	130	7	1	0	16
Leg, roasted, lean & fat	3 oz	230	15	0	0	23
lean only	3 oz	180	8	0	0	25
Light cure, roasted, lean & fat	3 oz	205	14	0	0	18
lean only	3 oz	135	5	0	0	21
Lunch meat, 1/8" slices	...	...	.	.	.	.
regular	2 slices	150	5	3	0	21
lean/ lowfat	2 slices	60	1	2	0	10
baked	2 slices	100	2	2	0	16
maple glazed	2 slices	120	2	6	Tr	18
smoked	2 slices	110	2	4	0	18
Hamburger & Cheeseburger	...	...	.	.	.	.
w/ catsup, mustard, lettuce,	...	...	.	.	.	.
& onion or pickle	...	...	.	.	.	.
4 oz burger w/o cheese	1	420	20	37	2	23
4 oz burger w/cheese	1	530	30	38	2	28
2 oz burger w/o cheese	1	260	9	32	2	14
2 oz burger w/cheese	1	340	15	35	2	16
(also, see Beef- Ground	...	...	.	.	.	.
& Fast Food Restaurants)	...	...	.	.	.	.
Hamburger Helper	...	...	.	.	.	.
Beef Pasta	1 cup	270	10	26	2	20
Beef Romanoff	1 cup	290	11	28	2	20
Beef Taco	1 cup	310	13	31	2	21
Beef Teriyaki	1 cup	290	10	34	2	18
Cheesy Shells	1 cup	340	14	30	2	22
Fettuccini Alfredo	1 cup	310	13	26	2	20
Zesty Italian	1 cup	320	11	34	2	21
Hash Browns – see Potatoes	...	...	.	.	.	.
Hearts of Palm, canned	1 piece	9	Tr	2	1	1
Honey	1 Tbsp	64	0	17	Tr	Tr
	1 cup	1030	0	279	1	1
Honeydew Melon	...	...	.	.	.	.
Fresh, avg size 6 ½" melon,	...	...	.	.	.	.
cubed or diced	1 cup	60	Tr	16	1	1
wedge, 1/8 of melon	1 wedge	55	Tr	15	1	1
Horseradish, as prep	1 tsp	4	Tr	1	Tr	Tr
HOT DOG (FRANKFURTER)	...	...	.	.	.	.
Beef or Pork	1	145	13	1	0	5
Chicken or Turkey	1	115	10	2	0	6
Lowfat, any meat	1	75	5	3	0	5

FOOD: (See Beverages & Fast Food Restaurants listed separately)	Serving Size	Cal-ories	Fat (g)	Carb (g)	Fi-ber (g)	Pro-tein (g)
Fat free, any meat	1	45	0	5	0	6
Hot Dog (meal as prep)	...	...	.	.	.	.
Hot Dog on Bun	...	...	.	.	.	.
w/ catsup & mustard	1 avg	245	15	19	1	10
Hot Dog on Bun w/ chili	1 avg	295	13	31	1	14
Corndog	1 avg	395	16	49	2	16
Hummus, commercial	1 Tbsp	23	1	2	1	1
Hush Puppies	5	260	12	35	2	5
Ice Cream	...	...	.	.	.	.
Chocolate	...	...	.	.	.	.
regular	½ cup	145	7	19	1	3
reduced fat	½ cup	100	3	15	1	3
Vanilla	...	...	.	.	.	.
regular	½ cup	135	7	16	0	2
reduced fat	½ cup	90	3	15	0	3
rich	½ cup	180	12	17	0	3
soft ice cream in cone	1 cone	200	13	19	0	4
soft in cone, chocolate dipped	1 cone	255	13	32	1	5
Sherbet, Orange	½ cup	100	1	22	0	1
Ice Cream Cone, 2 ½" cup only	1 cup	20	0	4	0	0
Ice Cream Sandwich, vanilla	1	220	9	31	1	4
Ice Pop - See Frozen Dessert	...	...	.	.	.	.
Italian Ices	½ cup	65	Tr	16	0	Tr
Italian Seasoning, dried spice	½ tsp	3	0	Tr	Tr	Tr
Jalapeno – see Peppers	...	...	.	.	.	.
Jam	...	...	.	.	.	.
All flavors, regular	1 Tbsp	55	Tr	14	Tr	Tr
All flavors, restaurant packet	1 pkt	39	Tr	10	Tr	Tr
Jello – see Gelatin	...	...	.	.	.	.
Jelly	...	...	.	.	.	.
All flavors, regular	1 Tbsp	54	Tr	13	Tr	Tr
All flavors, restaurant packet	1 pkt	40	Tr	10	Tr	Tr
Kale	...	...	.	.	.	.
Fresh, raw	1 cup	17	Tr	4	2	1
Fresh, chopped, cooked	1 cup	36	Tr	7	3	2
Frozen, chopped, cooked	1 cup	39	Tr	7	3	3
Ketchup, regular	1 Tbsp	18	Tr	4	Tr	Tr
restaurant size packet	1 pkt	10	Tr	3	Tr	Tr
Kiwi fruit, fresh, medium size	1	45	Tr	11	3	1
Knockwurst, beef, Boars Head	1 wurst	310	27	1	Tr	15

FOOD: (See Beverages & Fast Food Restaurants listed separately)	Serving Size	Cal-ories	Fat (g)	Carb (g)	Fi-ber (g)	Pro-tein (g)
Kohlrabi, cooked, slices	1 cup	48	Tr	11	2	3
Lamb	...	...	.	.	.	.
(Braised, broiled, or roasted)	...	...	.	.	.	.
Arm chop, lean & fat	3 oz	295	20	0	0	26
lean only	3 oz	235	12	0	0	30
Leg of lamb, lean & fat	3 oz	220	14	0	0	22
lean only	3 oz	160	7	0	0	24
Loin chop, lean & fat	3 oz	270	20	0	0	21
lean only	3 oz	185	8	0	0	25
Rib roast, lean & fat	3 oz	305	25	0	0	18
lean only	3 oz	195	11	0	0	22
Lard	1 cup	1850	205	0	0	0
	1 Tbsp	115	13	0	0	0
Lasagna, avg size 2 ½" x 4 "	...	...	.	.	.	.
w/ meat sauce	1	360	12	52	2	18
w/ zucchini	1	330	2	58	3	20
Leek, chopped, cooked	1 cup	32	Tr	8	1	1
Lemon, fresh, 2 ¼" dia	1	20	Tr	4	2	1
Lentil, cooked	½ cup	115	1	20	8	9
Lettuce, fresh, raw	...	...	.	.	.	.
Bibb, Boston, Butterhead	...	...	.	.	.	.
whole head, 5" dia	1 head	21	Tr	4	2	2
single leaf	1 leaf	1	Tr	Tr	Tr	Tr
Iceberg, Crisphead	...	.	Tr	.	.	.
whole head, 6" dia	1 head	65	1	11	8	5
single leaf	1 leaf	1	Tr	Tr	Tr	Tr
pieces, chopped or shredded	1 cup	8	Tr	1	Tr	1
wedge slice, 1/6 of 6" head	1 wedge	11	Tr	2	1	1
Loose leaf	...	...	.	.	.	.
single leaf	1 leaf	2	Tr	Tr	Tr	Tr
pieces, shredded or chopped	1 cup	10	Tr	2	1	1
Romaine or cos	...	...	.	.	.	.
innerleaf	1 leaf	1	Tr	Tr	Tr	Tr
pieces, shredded	1 cup	8	Tr	1	Tr	1
Lime, fresh, 2" dia	1	20	Tr	5	2	Tr
Linguini w/Clam sauce	...	...	.	.	.	.
Lean Cuisine entrée	1 meal	260	7	32	2	16
Liver	...	...	.	.	.	.
Beef liver, fried	3 oz	185	7	7	0	23
Chicken liver, simmered	1 liver	31	1	Tr	0	5
Veal liver, braised	3.5 oz	165	7	0	0	22

FOOD: (See Beverages & Fast Food Restaurants listed separately)	Serving Size	Cal- ories	Fat (g)	Carb (g)	Fi- ber (g)	Pro- tein (g)
Liverwurst, Boars Head	2 oz	170	15	1	Tr	8
Lobster – see Fish / Seafood	...	...	.	.	.	.
Lo Mein w/Vegetables	1 ½ cup	230	4	40	3	8
Lo Mein w/meat & vegetables	1 ½ cup	310	12	35	1	13
Lunch Meat (thin 1/8" slices)	...	...	.	.	.	.
Beef or Pork, regular	2 slices	180	16	2	0	7
Beef or Pork, lowfat	2 slices	110	9	2	0	6
Beef or Pork, fat free	2 slices	60	1	3	0	8
Chicken or Turkey , regular	2 slices	160	14	2	0	7
Chicken or Turkey, lowfat	2 slices	100	8	2	0	6
Chicken or Turkey, fat free	2 slices	60	1	3	0	8
Ham, regular	2 slices	150	5	3	0	21
Ham, lean/lowfat	2 slices	60	1	2	0	10
(also see specific listings)	...	.	.	.	.	.
Macaroni, elbows	...	...	.	.	.	.
Dry, uncooked	1 cup	420	2	82	4	14
Plain, cooked	1 cup	195	1	40	2	7
Macaroni & Cheese	1 cup	300	10	40	3	10
Mackerel – see Fish	...	...	.	.	.	.
Malt O Meal, as prep	1 cup	122	Tr	26	1	4
Mandarin Oranges	...	...	.	.	.	.
Canned in light syrup	1 cup	154	Tr	41	2	1
Mango	...	...	.	.	.	.
Fresh, peeled, 11 oz	1 mango	135	1	35	4	1
Fresh, peeled, sliced	1 cup	105	Tr	28	3	1
Manicotti, 3 cheese	2 piece	300	9	40	1	16
Margarine	...	...	.	.	.	.
Regular, 4 sticks/Lb	1 stick	815	90	1	0	1
Regular, hard or soft	1 cup	1625	185	1	0	2
Regular, hard or soft	1 Tbsp	100	11	Tr	0	Tr
Regular, hard or soft	1 tsp	34	4	Tr	0	Tr
Reduced fat 50%	1 cup	1235	139	0	0	1
Reduced fat 50%	1 tsp	25	3	0	0	Tr
Fat free	1 cup	512	Tr	0	0	Tr
Fat free	1 Tbsp	5	0	0	0	0
Spread or blend type, regular	1 Tbsp	100	11	Tr	0	Tr
Spread or blend w/ vegetable oil & margarine, 33% reduced fat	1 Tbsp	60	7	0	0	0
Marjoram, dried spice	1 tsp	2	0	Tr	Tr	Tr
Marmalade	1 Tbsp	50	Tr	14	Tr	Tr

FOOD: (See Beverages & Fast Food Restaurants listed separately)	Serving Size	Cal-ories	Fat (g)	Carb (g)	Fi-ber (g)	Pro-tein (g)
Marshmallow	...	...	.	.	.	.
Miniature size	1 cup	160	Tr	41	Tr	Tr
Regular size	2 piece	46	Tr	12	Tr	Tr
Regular or Large size	1 oz	90	Tr	23	Tr	Tr
Marshmallow Topping	1 Tbsp	50	Tr	12	Tr	Tr
Mayonnaise	...	...	.	.	.	.
Regular	1 Tbsp	100	11	Tr	0	Tr
Light / reduced calorie	1 Tbsp	50	5	1	0	Tr
Fat free	1 Tbsp	10	0	2	0	Tr
Meat – see specific listings	...	...	.	.	.	.
Meat Tenderizer	¼ tsp	0	0	0	0	0
Meatless Burger	...	...	.	.	.	.
Single patty, broiled	1 patty	100	1	9	4	15
Cooked, crumbled	1 cup	230	13	7	5	22
Meatloaf	...	...	.	.	.	.
Banquet entrée	1 meal	280	16	22	1	13
Healthy Choice entrée	1 meal	320	5	52	1	15
Lean Cuisine entrée	1 meal	260	7	28	1	20
Meatloaf & cheese sandwich	1	350	13	41	2	18
Minestrone – see Soup	...	...	.	.	.	.
Molasses, blackstrap	1 Tbsp	47	0	12	0	0
	1 cup	771	0	199	0	0
Mortadella	1 slice	50	4	Tr	0	2
Muffin	...	...	.	.	.	.
Avg size muffin, 2 ½" dia	...	...	.	.	.	.
Apple	1	160	4	28	2	3
Banana	1	165	4	29	2	3
Blueberry	1	160	4	28	2	3
Bran w/ raisins	1	175	5	36	4	4
Chocolate Chip	1	180	5	37	2	3
Corn	1	175	5	29	2	3
Extra large muffin, 4" dia	...	...	.	.	.	.
Banana nut	1	420	11	75	8	7
Bran w/raisins	1	425	11	76	8	8
(also see English Muffin)	...	...	.	.	.	.
Mulberries	½ cup	30	Tr	7	3	Tr
Mushroom	...	...	.	.	.	.
Regular Mushrooms	...	...	.	.	.	.
Fresh, raw, slices	1 cup	18	Tr	3	1	2
Fresh, sliced, cooked	1 cup	42	Tr	8	3	3
Canned, stems & pieces, cooked	1 cup	37	Tr	8	4	3

FOOD: (See Beverages & Fast Food Restaurants listed separately)	Serving Size	Cal- ories	Fat (g)	Carb (g)	Fi- ber (g)	Pro- tein (g)
Shiitake Mushrooms	...	...	.	.	.	.
Dried, cut pieces, cooked	1 cup	80	Tr	20	3	2
Dried, whole, cooked	1 whole	11	Tr	3	Tr	Tr
Mussels – see Fish/Seafood	...	...	.	.	.	.
Mustard, yellow	...	...	.	.	.	.
Regular	1 tsp	4	Tr	Tr	Tr	Tr
Hot or Honey flavored	1 tsp	8	Tr	2	Tr	Tr
Powder	1 tsp	10	Tr	2	Tr	Tr
Mustard Greens	...	...	.	.	.	.
Chopped, cooked	1 cup	21	Tr	3	2	3

FOODS: N through Z

FOOD: (See Beverages & Fast Food Restaurants listed separately)	Serving Size	Cal- ories	Fat (g)	Carb (g)	Fi- ber (g)	Pro- tein (g)
Nachos w/ Cheese sauce	7 pieces	345	19	36	3	9
Nectarine, fresh, med, 2 ½" dia	1	67	1	16	2	1
Noodles (egg noodles)	...	...	.	.	.	.
Dry, uncooked	1 cup	420	2	82	4	14
Plain, cooked	1 cup	195	1	40	2	7
Chow Mein noodles, dry crunchy	1 cup	235	14	26	2	4
Spinach noodles, cooked	1 cup	210	3	39	4	8
Noodles Alfredo	¾ cup	250	7	39	2	10
Noodles Stroganoff	¾ cup	220	4	37	2	9
Nut Pastry Filling	1 Tbsp	65	2	13	1	2
Nuts	...	...	.	.	.	.
Almonds	...	...	.	.	.	.
sliced almonds	1 cup	550	48	19	11	20
whole almonds, about 24	1 oz	165	14	6	3	6
Brazil nuts, shelled, 6 to 8 nuts	1 oz	185	19	4	2	4
Cashews	...	...	.	.	.	.
dry roasted, about 20	1 oz	160	13	9	1	4
oil roasted, about 18	1 oz	165	14	8	1	5
Chestnuts, roasted, shelled	1 cup	350	3	76	7	5
Coconut	...	...	.	.	.	.
fresh, shredded	1 cup	285	27	12	7	3
dried, sweetened flakes	1 cup	465	33	44	4	3

FOOD: (See Beverages & Fast Food Restaurants listed separately)	Serving Size	Cal-ories	Fat (g)	Carb (g)	Fi-ber (g)	Pro-tein (g)
Hazelnuts, chopped, ¼ cup	1 oz	180	17	5	3	4
Macadamia, dry roasted, 11 nuts	1 oz	205	22	4	2	2
Mixed Nuts w/ peanuts	...	...	.	.	.	.
dry roasted, about 20 nuts	1 oz	168	15	7	3	5
oil roasted, about 20 nuts	1 oz	175	16	6	3	5
Peanuts	...	...	.	.	.	.
dry roasted, unsalted	1 cup	855	73	31	12	35
dry roasted, unsalted, about 28	1 oz	165	14	6	2	7
dry roasted, salted, about 28	1 oz	165	14	6	2	7
honey roasted, about 28	1 oz	165	13	7	2	7
oil roasted, salted, about 26	1 oz	170	15	5	3	7
Pecans, 10 whole or 20 halves	1 oz	195	20	4	3	3
Pine nuts, shelled	1 oz	160	14	4	1	7
Pistachio nuts, dry roasted,	...	...	.	.	.	.
shelled, about 47	1 oz	160	13	8	3	6
Walnuts, English	...	...	.	.	.	.
chopped	1 cup	785	78	16	8	18
whole, 7 walnuts	1 oz	185	18	4	2	4
Oat Bran	...	...	.	.	.	.
Uncooked	1 cup	230	7	62	15	16
Cooked	1 cup	88	2	25	6	7
Oatmeal, as prep	...	...	.	.	.	.
Plain, sweetened	½ cup	75	1	13	2	3
Fruit flavored oatmeal	1 pkt	135	2	26	2	3
Maple & brown sugar oatmeal	1 pkt	130	1	27	6	3
Oats, dry, 100% rolled oats	½ cup	150	3	26	4	5
OIL (for cooking & salads)	...	...	.	.	.	.
Cooking spray, ¼ second spray	1 spray	0	0	0	0	0
Canola oil	1 cup	1925	218	0	0	0
Canola oil	Tbsp	120	14	0	0	0
Corn oil	1 cup	1925	218	0	0	0
Corn oil	Tbsp	120	14	0	0	0
Cottonseed/soybean oil blend	1 cup	1925	218	0	0	0
Cottonseed/soybean oil blend	1 Tbsp	120	14	0	0	0
Olive oil	1 cup	1905	216	0	0	0
Olive oil	1 Tbsp	119	14	0	0	0
Peanut oil	1 cup	1905	216	0	0	0
Peanut oil	1 Tbsp	119	14	0	0	0
Safflower oil	1 cup	1925	218	0	0	0
Safflower oil	1 Tbsp	120	14	0	0	0
Sesame oil	1 cup	1925	218	0	0	0

FOOD: (See Beverages & Fast Food Restaurants listed separately)	Serving Size	Cal- ories	Fat (g)	Carb (g)	Fi- ber (g)	Pro- tein (g)
Sesame oil	1 Tbsp	120	14	0	0	0
Soybean oil	1 cup	1925	218	0	0	0
Soybean oil	1 Tbsp	120	14	0	0	0
Sunflower oil	1 cup	1925	218	0	0	0
Sunflower oil	1 Tbsp	120	14	0	0	0
Vegetable oil	1 cup	1925	218	0	0	0
Vegetable oil	1 Tbsp	120	14	0	0	0
Okra	...	...	.	.	.	.
Fresh, sliced, cooked	1 cup	51	Tr	12	4	3
Frozen, slices, cooked	1 cup	52	1	11	5	4
Whole, 3" pods, cooked	8 pods	30	Tr	7	2	2
Fried, breaded	½ cup	165	10	17	4	3
Olive	...	...	.	.	.	.
Pickled, green, medium size	5	20	2	Tr	Tr	Tr
Ripe, black, large size	5	25	2	1	Tr	Tr
Olive Loaf	2 oz	130	12	1	Tr	6
Onion	...	...	.	.	.	.
Round yellow or white onion	...	...	.	.	.	.
Fresh, raw, whole, 2 ½" dia	1 whole	42	Tr	9	2	1
Fresh, chopped	1 cup	61	Tr	14	3	2
Fresh, sliced, 1/8" thick	1 slice	5	Tr	1	Tr	Tr
Cooked, whole, 2 ½" dia	1 whole	41	Tr	10	1	1
Cooked, sliced or chopped	1 cup	92	Tr	21	3	3
Sprigs w/green tops & bulbs	...	...	.	.	.	.
Whole w/top, raw, chopped	1 whole	8	Tr	1	Tr	1
Bulbs only, chopped	1 cup	32	Tr	7	3	2
Onion Flakes, dried	1 Tbsp	16	Tr	4	Tr	Tr
Onion Powder or Salt	1 tsp	7	Tr	2	Tr	Tr
Onion Rings	...	...	.	.	.	.
Breaded, fried	5 rings	125	7	13	1	2
Orange	...	...	.	.	.	.
Fresh, medium size, 3" dia	1	70	Tr	15	3	1
Fresh, sections	1 cup	85	Tr	20	4	2
Oregano, ground	1 tsp	5	Tr	1	Tr	Tr
Pam, non-stick cooking spray	...	...	.	.	.	.
¼ second spray	1 spray	0	0	0	0	0
Pancake, 4" dia	...	...	.	.	.	.
Regular, toaster type	1	82	1	16	1	2
Lowfat, toaster type	1	70	Tr	17	1	2
Regular, from mix or scratch	1	90	2	17	1	2
Blueberry, mix or toaster type	1	85	1	15	1	2

FOOD: (See Beverages & Fast Food Restaurants listed separately)	Serving Size	Cal-ories	Fat (g)	Carb (g)	Fi-ber (g)	Pro-tein (g)
Pancake Syrup - see Syrup	...	...	.	.	.	.
Papaya	...	...	.	.	.	.
Fresh, peeled, 5" long x 3" dia	1	120	Tr	30	6	2
Fresh, peeled, cubed	1 cup	55	Tr	14	3	1
Paprika, dried powder	1 tsp	6	Tr	1	Tr	Tr
Parsley	...	...	.	.	.	.
Fresh, raw, chopped	10	4	Tr	1	Tr	Tr
Dried parsley bits	1 Tbsp	4	Tr	1	Tr	Tr
Parsnip, sliced, cooked	1 cup	125	Tr	30	6	2
Passion Fruit, raw, avg size	1	17	Tr	4	Tr	Tr
Pasta	...	...	.	.	.	.
Plain, cooked	1 cup	195	1	40	2	7
W/cheese & tomato sauce	1 cup	250	6	41	3	7
W/meatballs in tomato sauce	1 cup	260	10	31	3	11
W/shrimp & herb sauce	1 cup	295	10	40	3	10
W/tomato sauce	1 cup	240	5	41	3	7
Pasta Roni	...	...	.	.	.	.
Pasta w/broccoli	1 cup	240	4	37	3	7
Pasta w/broccoli & chicken	1 cup	260	5	37	3	8
Pasta Alfredo Primavera	1 cup	280	7	44	3	11
Pasta, Angel Hair	...	...	.	.	.	.
Prep w/herb sauce	1 cup	280	9	42	3	7
Weight Watchers entrée	1 meal	170	2	29	2	8
Pasta, Bowtie w/tomato sauce	1 cup	240	5	41	3	7
Pasta Marsala	1 cup	280	9	36	3	13
Pasta Salad w/dressing	1 cup	250	10	32	2	5
Pastrami	...	...	.	.	.	.
Regular	2 oz	90	4	2	Tr	12
Turkey	2 oz	60	1	1	Tr	13
Pastry - see Danish Pastry & specific listings	...	...	.	.	.	.
	...	...	.	.	.	.
Pastry Filling -see specific listing	...	...	.	.	.	.
Peach	...	...	.	.	.	.
Fresh, whole, med, 2 ½" dia	1	42	Tr	11	2	1
Fresh, sliced	1 cup	76	Tr	19	3	1
Canned, in heavy syrup	1 cup	195	Tr	52	3	1
Canned, in light syrup	1 cup	150	Tr	39	2	1
Canned, in juice	1 cup	115	Tr	28	3	2
Dried, halves,	3 halves	93	Tr	24	3	1
Frozen, sweetened slices, thawed	1 cup	235	Tr	60	5	2

FOOD: (See Beverages & Fast Food Restaurants listed separately)	Serving Size	Cal-ories	Fat (g)	Carb (g)	Fi-ber (g)	Pro-tein (g)
Peanut - see Nuts	...	...	.	.	.	.
Peanut Butter	...	...	.		.	.
Regular, smooth	1 Tbsp	95	8	3	1	4
Regular, chunky	1 Tbsp	95	8	3	1	4
Reduced fat, smooth	1 Tbsp	90	6	6	1	5
Pear	...	...	.	.	.	.
Fresh, 2 ½" dia	1	50	Tr	13	4	1
Fresh, 3 ¼" dia	1	116	1	29	9	1
Canned, in heavy syrup	1 cup	197	Tr	51	4	1
Canned, in juice	1 cup	125	Tr	32	4	1
Peas (cooked w/o fats)	...	...	.	.	.	.
Black eyed peas	½ cup	105	Tr	26	8	4
Chickpeas	½ cup	140	2	25	6	7
Green peas	½ cup	60	Tr	11	4	4
Lentils	½ cup	115	1	20	8	9
Navy peas	½ cup	125	1	24	6	8
Pea Pods	½ cup	40	Tr	7	2	3
Split peas	½ cup	115	1	20	8	8
Sweet peas	½ cup	60	Tr	11	4	4
Peas and Carrots	½ cup	40	Tr	8	3	3
Pecan Pastry Filling	1 Tbsp	65	2	13	1	2
Pecans, 10 whole or 20 halves	1 oz	195	20	4	3	3
Pepper, dried powder or granules	...	...	.	.	.	.
Black	1 tsp	5	Tr	1	Tr	Tr
Cayenne or red	1 tsp	7	Tr	1	Tr	Tr
White	1 tsp	5	Tr	1	Tr	Tr
Pepper Steak	...	...	.	.	.	.
Stouffer's entree	1 meal	330	9	45	1	17
Le Menu entree	1 meal	354	13	35	1	26
Pepperoni, 14 thin slices/oz	1 oz	130	12	0	0	6
Peppers	...	...	.	.	.	.
Chili Peppers, hot, raw	...	...	.	.	.	.
red or green	1 whole	18	Tr	4	1	1
Green, sweet, raw	...	...	.	.	.	.
whole, 3" x 2 ¼"	1 whole	32	Tr	8	2	1
ring, ¼" thick	1 ring	3	Tr	1	Tr	Tr
chopped	1 cup	40	Tr	10	3	1
Jalapeno peppers, sliced	¼ cup	7	Tr	1	Tr	Tr
Red, sweet, raw	...	...	.	.	.	.
whole, 3" x 2 ¼"	1 whole	32	Tr	8	2	1
ring, ¼" thick	1 ring	3	Tr	1	Tr	Tr

FOOD: (See Beverages & Fast Food Restaurants listed separately)	Serving Size	Cal-ories	Fat (g)	Carb (g)	Fi-ber (g)	Pro-tein (g)
chopped	1 cup	40	Tr	10	3	1
Red or Green, sweet, cooked	...	...	.	.	.	.
chopped	1 cup	38	Tr	9	2	1
Peppers, Stuffed, Stouffers	1 cup	200	5	27	3	11
Persimmon, raw, medium size	1	32	Tr	8	2	Tr
Pickle	...	...	.	.	.	.
Bread & Butter slices, 1 ½" dia	6 slices	36	Tr	8	1	Tr
Dill, whole, 3 ¾" long	1	12	Tr	3	1	Tr
Sweet Gherkin, 2 ½" long	1	20	Tr	5	Tr	Tr
Pickle Relish	1 Tbsp	20	Tr	5	Tr	Tr
Pie (1/8 of 9" pie unless noted)	...	...	.	.	.	.
Apple pie, 2 crust	1 slice	420	19	59	4	4
Blueberry pie, 2 crust	1 slice	360	17	49	4	4
Boston Cream Pie, 1 crust	1 slice	230	8	39	1	2
Cherry pie, 2 crust	1 slice	485	22	69	4	5
Cherry, fried pie, 4" x 2"	1 slice	405	21	55	3	4
Chocolate chip pie, 1 crust	1 slice	590	34	57	3	6
Chocolate Cream pie, 1 crust	1 slice	405	22	45	3	4
Coconut Custard pie, 1 crust	1 slice	305	15	36	2	7
Lemon Meringue pie, 1 crust	1 slice	360	16	50	1	5
Peach pie, 2 crust	1 slice	410	19	58	3	4
Pecan pie, 1 crust	1 slice	505	27	64	2	6
Pumpkin pie, 1 crust	1 slice	320	14	41	3	7
Strawberry pie, 2 crust	1 slice	360	16	50	2	5
Pie Crust, 9" dia	...	...	.	.	.	.
Regular from recipe or frozen	1 crust	800	50	75	2	9
Graham cracker crust	1 crust	950	51	110	3	9
Reduced fat crust	1 crust	605	30	74	2	8
Pilaf - see Rice Pilaf	...	...	.	.	.	.
Pimiento	1 oz	10	Tr	2	Tr	Tr
Pineapple	...	...	.	.	.	.
Fresh, diced or sliced	1 cup	76	1	19	2	1
Canned, in heavy syrup,	...	...	.	.	.	.
chunks or crushed	1 cup	198	Tr	51	2	1
slices, 3" dia	1 slice	38	Tr	10	Tr	Tr
Canned, in juice,	...	...	.	.	.	.
chunks or crushed	1 cup	150	Tr	39	2	1
slices, 3" dia	1 slice	28	Tr	7	1	Tr
PIZZA (Listings for an avg size	...	...	.	.	.	.
slice, 1/8 of 12" pizza)	...	...	.	.	.	.
Thin & Crispy Pizza	...	...	.	.	.	.

FOOD: (See Beverages & Fast Food Restaurants listed separately)	Serving Size	Cal- ories	Fat (g)	Carb (g)	Fi- ber (g)	Pro- tein (g)
Cheese	1 slice	140	3	21	1	8
Pepperoni & Cheese	1 slice	180	7	20	1	10
One Meat w/ Vegetables	1 slice	185	5	21	2	13
Three Meat w/ Vegetables	1 slice	210	9	21	2	12
Thick & Chewy or Pan Pizza	...	...	.	.	.	.
Cheese	1 slice	270	6	39	1	15
Pepperoni & Cheese	1 slice	310	8	39	1	19
One Meat w/ Vegetables	1 slice	320	12	38	2	15
Three Meat w/ Vegetables	1 slice	405	17	40	2	24
Stuffed Crust Pizza, thick	...	...	.	.	.	.
Pepperoni & Cheese	1 slice	350	14	39	1	20
Three Meat w/ Vegetables	1 slice	450	21	40	2	21
Pizza Rolls, 1 ½", frozen, heated	...	...	.	.	.	.
With cheese and one meat	5 pieces	175	7	20	1	9
Plantain, without peel	...	...	.	.	.	.
Fresh, medium size	1	218	1	57	4	2
Cooked, slices	1 cup	180	Tr	48	4	1
Plum	...	...	.	.	.	.
Fresh, whole, med, 2 ¼" dia	1	36	Tr	9	1	1
Canned, in heavy syrup	1 cup	230	Tr	60	3	1
Canned, in juice	1 cup	146	Tr	38	3	1
Pomegranate, avg size, raw	1	105	1	26	2	2
Pop Tart – see Toaster Pastry	...	...	.	.	.	.
Popcorn	...	...	.	.	.	.
Air popped	1 cup	30	Tr	6	1	1
Caramel coated w/ peanuts	1 cup	170	3	34	2	3
Caramel coated w/o peanuts	1 cup	150	5	28	2	1
Cheese flavored	1 cup	60	4	6	1	1
Microwave, butter flavor	1 cup	40	2	4	1	1
Microwave, butter, reduced fat	1 cup	30	1	5	1	1
Popped in oil	1 cup	55	3	6	1	1
Popped in oil, buttered	1 cup	75	5	6	1	1
Popcorn Cake, plain	1	38	Tr	8	Tr	1
Butter flavor	1	40	Tr	8	Tr	1
Carmel	1	48	Tr	11	Tr	1
Poppyseed pastry filling	1 Tbsp	65	1	14	1	1
Popsicle – see Frozen Dessert	...	...	.	.	.	.
PORK	...	...	.	.	.	.
(Weights for meat w/o bones)	...	...	.	.	.	.
Bacon, regular	3 slices	110	9	Tr	0	6
Bacon, Canadian	3 slices	125	6	1	0	17

FOOD: (See Beverages & Fast Food Restaurants listed separately)	Serving Size	Cal-ories	Fat (g)	Carb (g)	Fi-ber (g)	Pro-tein (g)
Boston Butt, roasted, lean	3 oz	205	9	0	0	27
Picnic Pork	3.5 oz	280	21	Tr	0	20
Pork Chop, loin cut	...	...	.	.	.	.
broiled, lean & fat	3 oz	205	11	0	0	24
broiled, lean only	3 oz	170	7	0	0	26
pan fried, lean & fat	3 oz	235	14	0	0	25
pan fried, lean only	3 oz	195	9	0	0	27
Rib Roast, lean & fat	3 oz	215	13	0	0	23
lean only	3 oz	195	9	0	0	24
Sausage	...	...	.	.	.	.
breakfast link, small	1 link	70	6	Tr	0	3
breakfast patty, small	1 patty	80	7	Tr	0	3
sausage, regular	2 oz	120	10	1	0	7
sausage, lowfat	2 oz	80	2	6	0	7
Polish Kielbasa sausage	2 oz	120	10	Tr	0	8
Vienna sausage, 2" links	2 links	90	8	Tr	0	4
Shoulder cut, braised, lean & fat	3 oz	280	20	0	0	24
lean only	3 oz	210	10	0	0	27
Spareribs, braised	3 oz	335	26	0	0	25
(Other Pork Products, see:	...	...	.	.	.	.
Bologna, Ham, Hot Dog,	...	...	.	.	.	.
Salami, & specific entrées)	...	...	.	.	.	.
Pork Chop, fried	...	...	.	.	.	.
Marie Callendar entrée	1 meal	550	27	50	2	26
Pork Rinds, about 1 cup	1 oz	155	9	0	0	17
Pot Pie, 4" dia, frozen, heated	...	...	.	.	.	.
Beef Pot Pie	1 pie	480	27	40	2	19
Chicken Pot Pie	1 pie	410	23	38	2	11
Turkey Pot Pie	1 pie	400	22	38	2	11
Pot Roast	...	...	.	.	.	.
Lean Cuisine entrée	1 meal	190	6	19	1	15
Marie Callender entrée	1 meal	250	6	31	1	17
Swanson entrée	1 meal	405	10	48	2	30
POTATO	...	...	.	.	.	.
(also see Sweet Potatoes)	...	...	.	.	.	.
Au Gratin Potatoes	1 cup	300	16	28	4	9
Baked potato, 4 ¾" x 2 ¼"	...	...	.	.	.	.
whole potato w/skin	1	220	Tr	51	5	5
whole potato w/o skin	1	145	Tr	34	2	3
Baked, & filled or topped,	...	...	.	.	.	.
large potato, 6" x 2 ½"	...	...	.	.	.	.

FOOD: (See Beverages & Fast Food Restaurants listed separately)	Serving Size	Cal-ories	Fat (g)	Carb (g)	Fi-ber (g)	Pro-tein (g)
bacon & cheese	1	530	18	78	5	17
broccoli & cheese	1	470	14	80	6	9
cheese	1	570	23	78	5	14
chili & cheese	1	620	24	83	5	20
sour cream & chives	1	390	6	73	6	7
Boiled potato, 2 ½" dia	...	...	.	.	.	.
peeled, whole potato	1	116	Tr	27	2	2
peeled, diced	1 cup	134	Tr	31	3	3
French Fries	...	...	.	.	.	.
Frozen, heated	...	...	.	.	.	.
thin shoestring strips, 3 oz	20 fries	130	4	22	2	2
thick or crinkle cut, 4.5 oz	20 fries	195	6	33	3	3
Restaurant type, medium order	1 med	350	15	48	5	5
Hash Browns, patty, 3" x 2"	1 patty	80	9	9	1	2
Hash Browned potatoes	1 cup	280	14	32	2	4
Mashed, w/milk & margarine	1 cup	220	9	35	4	4
Scalloped potatoes	1 cup	245	11	29	4	8
Tater Tots type fried potatoes	10	175	8	24	3	3
Potato Chips	...	...	.	.	.	.
(about 14 chips, unless noted)	...	...	.	.	.	.
Plain, regular	1 oz	155	10	15	1	2
Barbecue flavor	1 oz	155	10	15	1	2
Cheddar cheese	1 oz	160	10	15	1	2
Fat free chips	1 oz	75	Tr	17	1	2
Pringles, regular	1 oz	160	11	15	1	1
Reduced fat chips	1 oz	140	7	18	1	2
Rippled chips (about 12 chips)	1 oz	160	10	15	1	2
Ruffles, original (12 chips)	1 oz	160	10	14	1	2
Ruffles, reduced fat (13 chips)	1 oz	150	7	18	1	2
Ranch flavor chips	1 oz	155	10	15	2	2
Sour cream & onion flavor	1 oz	155	10	15	2	2
Potato Salad	1 cup	360	21	28	3	7
Potato Sticks, fried, crunchy	1 cup	250	15	26	3	3
Preserves	...	...	.	.	.	.
All flavors, regular	1 Tbsp	55	Tr	14	Tr	Tr
All flavors, restaurant packet	1 pkt	39	Tr	10	Tr	Tr
Pretzels	...	...	.	.	.	.
Sticks, regular	25	58	1	12	1	1
Mini Twists, regular	10	58	1	12	1	1
Bavarian, twisted, 2 ½" x 3"	1	60	1	13	1	1
Chocolate coated	1 oz	130	5	20	1	2

FOOD: (See Beverages & Fast Food Restaurants listed separately)	Serving Size	Cal-ories	Fat (g)	Carb (g)	Fi-ber (g)	Pro-tein (g)
Dutch, twisted, 2 ½" x 3"	1	60	1	13	1	1
Honey Mustard nuggets	10	150	4	24	1	3
Soft, twisted, large, 3" x 5"	1	180	2	36	2	5
Sourdough, twisted, 2 ½" x 3"	1	60	1	13	1	1
Prosciutto, Boars Head	1 oz	60	3	0	0	8
Prunes, dried, pitted	…	…	.	.	.	.
Uncooked, unsweetened	5 prunes	100	Tr	26	3	1
Stewed, unsweetened	1 cup	265	1	70	16	3
Pudding	…	…	…	…	…	…
Butterscotch, regular	½ cup	150	5	25	Tr	3
Caramel w/chocolate, regular	½ cup	150	5	25	1	3
Chocolate, regular	½ cup	150	5	25	1	3
fat free	½ cup	105	Tr	23	1	3
sugar free	½ cup	110	1	18	1	2
Rice pudding, regular	½ cup	185	8	25	Tr	2
Tapioca, regular	½ cup	135	4	22	Tr	2
fat free	½ cup	100	Tr	23	Tr	2
Vanilla, regular	½ cup	145	4	25	Tr	3
fat free	½ cup	105	Tr	24	Tr	2
sugar free	½ cup	110	1	18	Tr	2
Pumpkin	…	…	.	.	.	.
Fresh, cooked, mashed	1 cup	50	Tr	12	3	2
Canned, heated	1 cup	83	1	20	7	3
Quesadilla	…	…	.	.	.	.
Cheese	1	350	18	31	2	16
Chicken	1	400	19	33	2	25
Radish, fresh, raw, avg 1" dia	5	5	Tr	1	Tr	Tr
Raisin	…	…	.	.	.	.
Golden or natural, not packed	1 cup	435	1	115	6	5
Golden or natural, 0.5 oz pkg	1 pkg	42	Tr	11	1	Tr
Golden or natural, not packed	3 Tbsp	84	Tr	22	1	Tr
Raisin Bran – see Cereal	…	…	.	.	.	.
Raspberries	…	…	.	.	.	.
Fresh	1 cup	60	1	14	8	1
Frozen, sweetened, thawed	1 cup	260	Tr	65	11	2
Ravioli	…	…	.	.	.	.
Beef	1 cup	255	4	44	1	12
Cheese	1 cup	265	5	44	1	11
Relish – see Pickle Relish or specific listing	… …	… …	. .	. .	. .	. .
Rhubarb	…	…	.	.	.	.

FOOD: (See Beverages & Fast Food Restaurants listed separately)	Serving Size	Cal- ories	Fat (g)	Carb (g)	Fi- ber (g)	Pro- tein (g)
Fresh, diced	1 cup	28	Tr	6	Tr	Tr
Frozen, cooked, sweetened	1 cup	278	Tr	75	5	1
RICE	...	...	.	.	.	.
Plain Rice Dishes	...	...	.	.	.	.
Brown long grain rice, boiled	1 cup	215	2	45	4	5
Brown long grain, prep w/butter	1 cup	315	13	45	4	5
Long grain & wild rice, boiled	1 cup	200	1	40	3	6
Long grain & wild prep w/butter	1 cup	300	12	40	3	6
White rice, boiled	1 cup	200	Tr	44	1	4
White rice, prep w/butter	1 cup	300	11	44	1	4
Wild rice, boiled	1 cup	170	1	35	3	7
Wild rice, prep w/butter	1 cup	270	12	35	3	7
Yellow rice, boiled	1 cup	220	Tr	49	3	5
Mixed & Flavored Rice Dishes	...	...	.	.	.	.
Flavored w/ beef or pork	1 cup	280	4	52	3	8
Fried rice w/ beef	1 cup	295	7	48	3	10
Fried rice w/ chicken	1 cup	265	6	44	3	9
Fried rice w/ pork	1 cup	290	6	48	3	11
Fried rice w/ shrimp	1 cup	260	5	44	3	9
Fried rice w/ vegetables	1 cup	255	4	48	3	7
Rice & beans	1 cup	300	7	49	3	11
Rice & vegetables	1 cup	260	3	50	3	8
Rice Pilaf w/vegetables	1 cup	240	3	45	3	6
Rice-a-Roni	...	...	.	.	.	.
Beef vermicelli rice dish	1 cup	290	4	51	3	9
Broccoli & cheddar rice dish	1 cup	330	8	48	3	10
Cheddar & herbs rice dish	1 cup	310	7	48	3	10
Chicken & vegetable rice	1 cup	290	3	51	3	8
Chicken vermicelli rice dish	1 cup	290	3	52	3	9
Herb & butter rice dish	1 cup	280	4	53	3	8
Mexican style rice	1 cup	265	4	45	3	7
Rice pilaf	1 cup	305	4	54	3	8
Spanish rice dish	1 cup	270	4	45	3	7
Rice Cake, plain	1	35	Tr	7	Tr	1
Butter flavor	1	40	Tr	8	Tr	1
Carmel	1	48	Tr	11	Tr	1
Rice Krispies Treat	1 bar	90	2	18	Tr	1
Rigatoni, meat sauce	...	...	.	.	.	.
Lean Cuisine entrée	1 meal	260	10	25	2	18
Roast Beef – see Beef	...	...	.	.	.	.
Roast Beef Sandwich	...	...	.	.	.	.

FOOD: (See Beverages & Fast Food Restaurants listed separately)	Serving Size	Cal-ories	Fat (g)	Carb (g)	Fi-ber (g)	Pro-tein (g)
3 oz meat w/ sauce	1 avg	390	19	33	3	23
Rolls – see Bread	...	...	.	.	.	.
Rosemary, dried spice	½ tsp	2	0	Tr	Tr	Tr
Rutabaga, cubed, cooked	1 cup	65	Tr	15	3	2
Saccharin sweetener	1 pkt	0	0	Tr	0	0
Sage, dried spice	½ tsp	1	0	Tr	Tr	Tr
SALAD DRESSING	...	...	.	.	.	.
Blue cheese, regular	1 Tbsp	75	8	1	0	1
Blue cheese, low calorie	1 Tbsp	15	1	1	0	1
Buttermilk, regular	1 Tbsp	60	6	1	0	Tr
Buttermilk, low calorie	1 Tbsp	15	1	1	0	Tr
Caesar, regular	1 Tbsp	80	8	Tr	Tr	Tr
Caesar, low calorie	1 Tbsp	17	1	3	Tr	Tr
French, regular	1 Tbsp	70	6	3	0	Tr
French, low calorie	1 Tbsp	25	1	4	0	Tr
Honey Dijon, regular	1 Tbsp	70	6	3	0	Tr
Honey Dijon, fat free	1 Tbsp	25	1	4	0	Tr
Italian, regular	1 Tbsp	70	7	1	0	Tr
Italian, low calorie	1 Tbsp	16	1	1	0	Tr
Mayonnaise, regular	1 Tbsp	100	11	Tr	0	Tr
Mayonnaise, light	1 Tbsp	50	5	1	0	Tr
Mayonnaise, fat free	1 Tbsp	10	0	2	0	Tr
Ranch, regular	1 Tbsp	70	6	2	0	Tr
Ranch, low calorie	1 Tbsp	20	1	3	0	Tr
Russian, regular	1 Tbsp	75	8	2	0	Tr
Russian, low calorie	1 Tbsp	25	1	4	Tr	Tr
Thousand island, regular	1 Tbsp	65	6	2	0	Tr
Thousand island, low calorie	1 Tbsp	26	2	2	Tr	Tr
Zero Carb Salad Dressing	...	...	.	.	.	.
Nature's Flavors	...	...	.	.	.	.
Carbfree Blue Cheese	2 Tbsp	30	3	0	0	1
Carbfree French	2 Tbsp	30	3	0	0	1
Salad, Tossed	...	...	.	.	.	.
All Vegetable salad, no dressing	1 ½ cup	60	Tr	11	4	3
Salad w/egg & cheese	...	...	.	.	.	.
no dressing	1 ½ cup	120	7	5	1	9
w/regular dressing, any type	1 ½ cup	200	17	6	1	10
w/light dressing, any type	1 ½ cup	135	7	9	1	9
Salad w/grilled chicken or turkey	...	...	.	.	.	.
no dressing	1 ½ cup	150	3	11	1	19
w/regular dressing, any type	1 ½ cup	250	13	12	1	20

FOOD: (See Beverages & Fast Food Restaurants listed separately)	Serving Size	Cal- ories	Fat (g)	Carb (g)	Fi- ber (g)	Pro- tein (g)
w/light dressing, any type (Also see Pasta Salad, Potato Salad, & other specific listings)	1 ½ cup	175	3 . .	15 . .	1 . .	19 . .
Salami	...	...	.	.	.	.
Regular, any meat	2 oz	130	11	1	0	7
Lowfat, Turkey or Chicken, thin 1/8" slices	... 2 slices	... 80	. 5	. 1	. 0	. 8
Cotto	2 slices	95	7	1	0	7
Dried type, 3" x 1/8" slices	2 slices	95	7	1	0	6
Hard	1 oz	110	9	1	0	6
Salisbury Steak	...	...	.	...	.	.
Banquet entrée	1 meal	220	16	8	1	9
Morton's entrée	1 meal	210	9	23	2	9
Stouffer's entrée	1 meal	240	15	10	1	17
Weight Watchers entrée	1 meal	150	9	24	1	19
Salsa	1 Tbsp	4	Tr	1	Tr	Tr
Salt	...	...	.	.	.	.
Regular	½ tsp	0	0	0	0	0
Reduced sodium	½ tsp	0	0	0	0	0
Seasoned	½ tsp	5	Tr	Tr	Tr	Tr
Sandwich, w/ 2.5 oz Meat on Lg 6 " bun, sub, or kaiser roll	... ...	... ...	. .	. .	. .	. .
Cold Cuts, mixed meats w/ sauce, cheese, tomato, lettuce	1 ...	455 ...	19 .	51 .	2 .	22 .
Ham & Cheese w/ sauce	1	550	21	57	4	33
Roast Beef w/ mayo, tomato, lettuce	. 1	. 410	. 13	. 44	. 2	. 29
Tuna salad w/ mayo, lettuce	1	585	28	55	2	30
Sandwich Meat – see Lunch Meat	...	...	.	.	.	.
Sandwich Spread	1 Tbsp	35	3	2	Tr	1
SAUCE	...	...	.	.	.	.
A1 Steak Sauce	1 Tbsp	15	0	3	Tr	0
Barbecue sauce, regular	1 Tbsp	20	Tr	4	1	Tr
Barbecue, thick or honey	1 Tbsp	40	1	8	Tr	Tr
Catsup	1 Tbsp	18	Tr	4	Tr	Tr
Cheese sauce	¼ cup	110	8	4	Tr	4
Chili sauce	¼ cup	60	Tr	13	3	1
Duck Sauce	1 Tbsp	20	0	4	Tr	0
Hoison sauce	1 Tbsp	35	1	7	Tr	1
Hollandaise sauce	1 Tbsp	18	1	2	Tr	1
Horseradish, prepared	1 tsp	4	Tr	1	Tr	Tr

FOOD: (See Beverages & Fast Food Restaurants listed separately)	Serving Size	Cal- ories	Fat (g)	Carb (g)	Fi- ber (g)	Pro- tein (g)
Hot sauce	1 tsp	1	Tr	Tr	Tr	Tr
Marinara sauce	¼ cup	36	1	5	1	1
Mayonnaise, regular	1 Tbsp	100	11	Tr	0	Tr
Mayonnaise, light	1 Tbsp	50	5	1	0	Tr
Mayonnaise, fat free	1 Tbsp	10	0	2	0	Tr
Mustard, regular	1 tsp	4	Tr	Tr	Tr	Tr
Mustard, hot or honey	1 tsp	8	Tr	2	Tr	Tr
Oyster sauce	1 Tbsp	5	Tr	1	Tr	Tr
Pasta sauce	¼ cup	35	1	5	1	1
Pepper sauce, hot	1 tsp	1	Tr	Tr	Tr	Tr
Pickle Relish	1 Tbsp	20	Tr	5	Tr	Tr
Pizza sauce	¼ cup	35	1	5	1	1
Salsa	1 Tbsp	4	Tr	1	Tr	Tr
Sloppy Joe sauce w/meat	1 Tbsp	45	2	5	1	2
Soy sauce	1 Tbsp	10	Tr	1	Tr	1
Spaghetti sauce	¼ cup	36	1	5	1	1
Steak Sauce	1 Tbsp	15	0	3	Tr	0
Sweet & Sour Sauce	1 Tbsp	20	0	4	Tr	0
Szechuan sauce	1 Tbsp	20	Tr	3	Tr	1
Tabasco sauce	1 tsp	1	Tr	Tr	Tr	Tr
Taco sauce	1 Tbsp	10	Tr	2	Tr	Tr
Tamari Sauce	1 Tbsp	11	0	1	0	2
Tartar sauce	1 Tbsp	45	4	2	Tr	0
Teriyaki sauce	1 Tbsp	20	Tr	4	Tr	1
Tomato sauce	½ cup	37	Tr	9	2	1
White sauce	¼ cup	92	6	6	Tr	3
Worcestershire sauce	1 Tbsp	12	0	3	Tr	0
Zero Carb Sauce	…	…	.	.	.	.
Nature's Flavors	…	…	.	.	.	.
Barbecue sauce	2 Tbsp	0	0	0	0	0
Honey Mustard sauce	2 Tbsp	0	0	0	0	0
Sauerkraut	1 cup	45	Tr	10	6	2
Sausage	…	…	.	.	.	.
Breakfast link, small	1 link	70	6	Tr	0	3
Breakfast patty, small	1 patty	80	7	Tr	0	3
Beef or Pork sausage	2 oz	120	10	1	0	7
Chicken or Turkey sausage	2 oz	98	8	1	0	6
Lowfat sausage, beef or pork	2 oz	80	2	6	0	7
Lowfat sausage, chicken or turkey	2 oz	78	2	6	0	7
Fat free sausage, beef or pork	2 oz	60	0	6	0	7
Fat free sausage,	…	…	.	.	.	.

78

FOOD: (See Beverages & Fast Food Restaurants listed separately)	Serving Size	Cal-ories	Fat (g)	Carb (g)	Fi-ber (g)	Pro-tein (g)
chicken or turkey	2 oz	58	0	6	0	7
Polish sausage, Kielbasa	2 oz	120	10	Tr	0	8
Vienna sausage, 2" links	2 links	90	8	Tr	0	4
Scallop - see Fish/Seafood	...	...	.	.	.	.
Seafood – see Fish/Seafood	...	...	.	.	.	.
Seasoning – see specific listings	...	...	.	.	.	.
Blended Seasoning w/ salt, garlic, onion, paprika, papain	... ½ tsp	... 2	. 0	. Tr	. Tr	. Tr
Seaweed	...	...	.	.	.	.
Kelp, raw	2 Tbsp	4	Tr	1	Tr	Tr
Spirulina, dried	1 Tbsp	3	Tr	Tr	Tr	1
Thin wrap sheets	1 sheet	10	Tr	2	Tr	1
Seeds	...	...	.	.	.	.
Pumpkin seeds, roasted	1 oz	148	12	4	1	9
Sesame seeds, plain	1 Tbsp	47	4	1	Tr	2
Sesame seeds, butter, roasted	1 Tbsp	90	8	3	1	3
Soybean seeds, dried, boiled	½ cup	145	7	9	5	15
Sunflower seeds, dry roasted	1 oz	165	14	7	3	5
(Also see specific listings)	...	...	.	.	.	.
Shallot, raw, chopped	1 Tbsp	7	Tr	2	Tr	Tr
Shark – see Fish	...	...	.	.	.	.
Sherbet, Orange	½ cup	100	1	22	0	1
Sherbet, Rainbow	½ cup	105	1	23	0	1
Shortening, regular cottonseed &	1 cup	1810	205	0	0	0
soybean blend	1 Tbsp	115	13	0	0	0
Shrimp – see Fish/Seafood & specific entrées	... ...	... ...	. .	. .	. .	. .
Shrimp & Broccoli w/creamy white sauce	... 1 cup	... 270	. 10	. 29	. 1	. 15
Shrimp & Pasta w/creamy white sauce	... 1 cup	... 300	. 13	. 34	. 1	. 14
Shrimp & Vegetables Hunan style	... 1 cup	... 240	. 7	. 30	. 3	. 14
Shrimp & Vegetables w/szechuan sauce	... 1 cup	... 230	. 6	. 30	. 3	. 14
Shrimp Marinara Weight Watchers entrée	... 1 meal	... 200	. 2	. 37	. 1	. 8
Sirloin Steak – see Beef	...	...	.	.	.	.
Snack Mix, Chex Mix	¾ cup	120	5	18	2	3
Sorbet, orange or raspberry	½ cup	120	0	30	0	0

FOOD: (See Beverages & Fast Food Restaurants listed separately)	Serving Size	Cal- ories	Fat (g)	Carb (g)	Fi- ber (g)	Pro- tein (g)
Soufflé, regular type	1 cup	250	20	3	1	12
SOUP (as prep)	...	...	.	.	.	.
Bouillon cube, regular,	...	...	.	.	.	.
all varieties, makes 1 cup	1 cube	5	Tr	1	Tr	Tr
Bouillon packet, low sodium,	...	...	.	.	.	.
all varieties, makes 1 cup	1 pkt	15	Tr	3	Tr	Tr
Broth, consommé, all varieties	1 cup	20	Tr	3	Tr	1
Bean w/ Ham soup	1 cup	185	7	24	9	8
Bean w/ Pork soup	1 cup	175	6	23	9	8
Beef Noodle soup	1 cup	83	3	9	1	5
Chicken Noodle soup, regular	1 cup	75	2	9	1	4
Chicken Noodle soup, chunky	1 cup	175	6	17	4	13
Chicken & Rice soup	1 cup	70	2	8	1	5
Chicken & Vegetable, regular	1 cup	90	1	12	1	6
Chicken & Vegetable, chunky	1 cup	165	5	19	1	12
Clam Chowder, Manhattan	1 cup	85	2	12	2	2
Clam Chowder, New England	1 cup	165	7	17	2	9
Clam Chowder, Low fat,	...	...	.	.	.	.
New England	1 cup	115	2	20	1	5
Cream of Broccoli soup	...	...	.	.	.	.
prep w/ water	1 cup	125	9	8	1	2
prep w/ milk	1 cup	195	14	14	1	6
Cream of Chicken soup	...	...	.	.	.	.
prep w/ water	1 cup	117	7	9	Tr	3
prep w/ milk	1 cup	190	11	15	Tr	7
Cream of Mushroom soup	...	...	.	.	.	.
prep w/ water	1 cup	130	9	9	1	2
prep w/ milk	1 cup	200	14	15	1	6
Lentil soup, low fat	1 cup	125	2	20	6	8
Minestrone	1 cup	85	3	11	1	4
Onion soup	1 cup	100	2	19	4	4
Pea soup	1 cup	160	3	26	3	9
Potato w/ bean soup	1 cup	170	7	23	2	6
Ramen Beef Noodle soup	1 cup	190	8	26	1	4
Ramen Chicken noodle soup	1 cup	190	8	26	1	4
Ramen Mushroom noodle soup	1 cup	180	7	26	1	4
Tomato soup, prep w/ water	1 cup	85	2	17	1	2
Tomato soup, prep w/ milk	1 cup	160	6	22	1	6
Vegetable soup	1 cup	72	2	12	1	2
Vegetable Beef soup	1 cup	90	2	11	1	7
Wisconsin Cheese soup	1 cup	280	18	20	2	10

FOOD: (See Beverages & Fast Food Restaurants listed separately)	Serving Size	Cal-ories	Fat (g)	Carb (g)	Fi-ber (g)	Pro-tein (g)
Sour cream	...	...	.	.	.	.
Regular	1 cup	495	48	10	0	7
Regular	1 Tbsp	25	3	1	0	Tr
Reduced fat	1 Tbsp	20	2	1	0	Tr
Fat free	1 Tbsp	12	0	2	0	Tr
Soy Burger, broiled	1 patty	100	1	9	3	15
Soybeans	...	...	.	.	.	.
dried mature seeds, cooked	½ cup	145	7	9	5	15
Spaghetti	...	...	.	.	.	.
Plain, cooked	1 cup	195	1	40	2	7
With cheese & tomato sauce	1 cup	220	2	41	3	8
With meatballs in tomato sauce	1 cup	240	4	41	3	7
With tomato sauce	1 cup	260	10	31	3	11
Spaghetti Bolognese, w/ meat sauce, Healthy Choice entrée	... 1 meal	... 255	. 3	. 43	. 5	. 14
Spare Ribs – see Pork	...	...	.	.	.	.
Spice – see specific listings	...	...	.	.	.	.
Blended Spice w/ basil, garlic, oregano, rosemary, thyme	... ½ tsp	... 3	. 0	. Tr	. Tr	. Tr
Spinach	...	...	.	.	.	.
Fresh, raw, chopped	1 cup	7	Tr	1	Tr	1
Fresh, chopped, cooked	1 cup	41	Tr	7	4	5
Frozen, chopped, cooked	1 cup	53	Tr	10	6	6
Canned, cooked	1 cup	50	Tr	7	5	6
Spinach Soufflé	1 cup	220	18	3	1	11
Spread	...	...	.	.	.	.
Cheese Spread	1 Tbsp	40	3	1	0	3
Sandwich Spread	1 Tbsp	35	3	2	Tr	1
(also see spreads in Margarine)	...	...	.	.	.	.
Squash	...	...	.	.	.	.
Butternut squash	¾ cup	150	6	25	4	2
Summer, raw, sliced	1 cup	23	Tr	5	2	1
Summer, cooked, slices	1 cup	36	1	8	3	2
Winter, baked, cubes	1 cup	80	1	18	6	2
Winter, frozen, cooked, mashed	1 cup	94	Tr	24	2	3
Squash Casserole	¾ cup	330	24	20	6	7
Steak – see Beef	...	...	.	.	.	.
Steak Sauce, A1	1 Tbsp	15	0	3	Tr	0
Strawberries	...	...	.	.	.	.
Fresh, medium size, 1 ¼" dia	10	40	Tr	9	3	1
Fresh, sliced	1 cup	50	1	12	4	1

FOOD: (See Beverages & Fast Food Restaurants listed separately)	Serving Size	Cal-ories	Fat (g)	Carb (g)	Fi-ber (g)	Pro-tein (g)
Frozen, sweetened, thawed	1 cup	245	Tr	66	5	1
Strawberry Shortcake	1 avg	275	15	20	2	6
Streusel (avg size slice)	...	...	.	.	.	.
Apple	1 slice	240	17	33	2	4
Cherry	1 slice	205	16	30	2	4
Stuffing, as prep	...	...	.	.	.	.
Traditional stuffing, seasoned,	...	...	.	.	.	.
meat flavored	1 cup	360	18	44	6	6
Corn bread stuffing, seasoned	1 cup	345	17	42	5	5
Succotash	½ cup	80	1	17	3	3
Sugar	...	...	.	.	.	.
White, regular, granulated	...	...	.	.	.	.
One cup	1 cup	774	0	200	0	0
One tablespoon	1 Tbsp	45	0	12	0	0
One teaspoon	1 tsp	15	0	4	0	0
Restaurant size packet	1 pkt	24	0	6	0	0
White, Confectioner's, Powdered	...	...	.	.	.	.
Unsifted, one cup	1 cup	31	0	8	0	0
Unsifted, one tablespoon	1 Tbsp	467	0	119	0	0
Brown Sugar	...	...	.	.	.	.
Packed, one cup	1 cup	827	0	214	0	0
Not packed , one cup	1 cup	545	0	141	0	0
Not packed, one tablespoon	1 Tbsp	34	0	9	0	0
Sugar Substitute	...	...	.	.	.	.
Aspartame sweetener	1 pkt	0	0	Tr	0	0
Saccharine sweetener	1 pkt	0	0	Tr	0	0
Sundae (small serving)	...	...	.	.	.	.
Hot Fudge	1	285	9	48	1	6
Strawberry	1	230	3	45	1	6
Strawberry Yogurt	1	275	1	59	1	9
Swedish Meatballs	...	...	.	.	.	.
Celentano, 6 meatball meal	1 meal	260	19	5	Tr	12
Lean Cuisine entrée	1 meal	290	7	35	1	22
Weight Watchers entrée	1 meal	290	7	34	1	18
Sweet 'N Low	1 pkt	0	0	Tr	0	0
Sweet Potato	...	...	.	.	.	.
Baked w/skin 4" x 2"	1 whole	165	Tr	38	4	3
Baked or Boiled w/o skin 4" x 2"	1 whole	150	Tr	35	3	3
Boiled, peeled, mashed	½ cup	170	3	30	3	3
Candied, 2 ½" x 2" pieces	1 piece	145	3	29	3	1

FOOD: (See Beverages & Fast Food Restaurants listed separately)	Serving Size	Cal- ories	Fat (g)	Carb (g)	Fi- ber (g)	Pro- tein (g)
Canned in syrup, drained	1 cup	210	1	50	6	3
Canned, vacuum pack, mashed	1 cup	230	1	54	5	4
Whipped, frozen, heated	½ cup	140	6	18	3	2
Sweet Potato Casserole	¾ cup	280	18	39	4	3
Sweet Roll - see specific listings	...	...	.	.	.	.
Syrup	...	...	.	.	.	.
Butterscotch	1 Tbsp	60	1	12	Tr	0
Chocolate, thin	1 Tbsp	55	Tr	12	Tr	Tr
Chocolate fudge, thick	1 Tbsp	65	2	12	1	1
Corn, light	1 Tbsp	56	0	15	0	0
Maple	1 Tbsp	52	Tr	13	0	0
Molasses, blackstrap	1 Tbsp	47	0	12	0	0
	1 cup	771	0	199	0	0
Pancake Syrup/Table Syrup	...	...	.	.	.	.
Regular	1 Tbsp	55	0	14	0	0
Light, reduced calorie	1 Tbsp	25	0	7	0	0
Sugar free	1 Tbsp	8	0	3	Tr	0
Zero Carb Syrup	...	...	.	.	.	.
Nature's Flavors	...	...	.	.	.	.
Apple	2 Tbsp	0	0	0	0	0
Brown Sugar	2 Tbsp	0	0	0	0	0
Chocolate	2 Tbsp	0	0	0	0	0
Maple	1 Tbsp	0	0	0	0	0
Taco (w/hard or soft shell)	...	...	.	.	.	.
Regular size, with beef	1	210	11	18	2	11
Regular size, with chicken	1	190	8	17	2	13
Large, with steak or beef	1	280	17	20	2	13
X-Lg, double decker, with beef	1	365	18	27	2	21
Taco Salad w/ ground beef, cheese, taco shell	... 1	... 275	. 15	. 24	. 2	. 13
Taco Shell (shell only)	...	...	.	.	.	.
Thin shell, 6" dia	1	60	3	8	1	1
Large shell	1	100	5	13	1	2
Tahini, from toasted kernels	1 Tbsp	90	8	3	1	3
Tamale, meatless	2 pieces	215	8	30	1	6
Beef, Swanson entrée	1 meal	350	13	46	1	13
Chicken, Swanson entrée	1 meal	325	12	45	1	8
Tangerine, fresh, med, 2 ½" dia	1	37	Tr	9	2	1
Tapioca, pearl, dry	1 cup	545	Tr	135	1	Tr
Taro Leaf, steamed	½ cup	18	Tr	4	2	1
Tarragon, ground	1 tsp	5	Tr	1	Tr	Tr

FOOD: (See Beverages & Fast Food Restaurants listed separately)	Serving Size	Cal-ories	Fat (g)	Carb (g)	Fi-ber (g)	Pro-tein (g)
Tater Tots fried potatoes	10	175	8	24	3	3
T-bone Steak – see Beef	...	...	.	.	.	.
Teriyaki – see Beef Teriyaki or Chicken Teriyaki	... ...	... ...	. .	. .	. .	. .
Thyme, dried spice	½ tsp	2	0	Tr	Tr	Tr
Toaster Pastry (Pop Tart)	...	...	.	.	.	.
Apple, frosted	1 pastry	200	5	37	1	2
Apple, unfrosted	1 pastry	185	5	34	1	2
Blueberry, frosted	1 pastry	200	5	37	1	2
Blueberry, unfrosted	1 pastry	185	5	34	1	2
Brown sugar, cinnamon, frosted	1 pastry	190	5	36	1	2
Chocolate, frosted	1 pastry	200	5	37	1	3
Chocolate fudge, frosted	1 pastry	200	5	36	1	3
Grape, frosted	1 pastry	200	5	37	1	2
Grape, unfrosted	1 pastry	185	5	34	1	2
Lowfat, frosted, any variety	1 pastry	170	2	37	1	2
Lowfat, unfrosted, any variety	1 pastry	155	2	33	1	2
S'mores, frosted	1 pastry	220	6	39	1	2
Strawberry, frosted	1 pastry	200	5	37	1	2
Strawberry, unfrosted	1 pastry	185	5	34	1	2
Tofu, plain, cooked, 4 oz	½ cup	80	4	2	Tr	9
Tomatillos, raw, medium size	2	22	Tr	4	1	Tr
Tomato	...	...	.	.	.	.
Fresh, raw, avg size 2 ½" dia	1 whole	26	Tr	6	1	1
Fresh, raw, cherry tomato	1 whole	4	Tr	1	Tr	Tr
Fresh, slices, ¼" thick	1 slice	4	Tr	1	Tr	Tr
Fresh, chopped or sliced	1 cup	38	1	8	2	2
Canned, liquids and solids	1 cup	46	Tr	10	2	2
Stewed, fresh or canned	1 cup	70	1	17	3	2
Sun Dried	...	...	.	.	.	.
Plain	1 piece	5	Tr	1	Tr	Tr
Packed in oil, drained	1 piece	6	Tr	1	Tr	Tr
Tomato Paste	1 cup	215	1	51	11	10
Tomato Puree	1 cup	100	Tr	24	5	4
Tomato Sauce	1 cup	74	Tr	18	3	3
Topping, for dessert	...	...	.	.	.	.
Butterscotch, regular	1 Tbsp	60	1	12	Tr	0
Butterscotch, light	1 Tbsp	30	Tr	8	Tr	0
Chocolate, regular	1 Tbsp	50	Tr	11	1	1
Chocolate, light	1 Tbsp	25	Tr	7	Tr	Tr
Cream, Whipped Topping	...	...	.	.	.	.

FOOD: (See Beverages & Fast Food Restaurants listed separately)	Serving Size	Cal- ories	Fat (g)	Carb (g)	Fi- ber (g)	Pro- tein (g)
Light cream	1 cup	700	75	7	0	5
Light cream	1 Tbsp	45	5	Tr	0	Tr
Heavy cream	1 cup	820	88	7	0	5
Heavy cream	1 Tbsp	50	6	Tr	0	Tr
Pressurized in can	1 Tbsp	8	1	Tr	0	Tr
Marshmallow Topping	1 Tbsp	50	Tr	12	Tr	Tr
Strawberry Topping	1 Tbsp	50	Tr	11	Tr	1
Tortellini	...	...	.	.	.	.
Cheese filling	1 cup	270	7	40	2	12
Meat filling	1 cup	340	9	55	1	21
Spinach filling	1 cup	235	5	30	2	12
Tortellini Salad w/dressing	¾ cup	350	24	24	5	11
Tortilla, 6" dia, ready to cook	...	...	.	.	.	.
Corn	1	60	1	12	1	1
Flour	1	105	2	18	1	3
Tortilla Chips	...	...	.	.	.	.
Regular	1 oz	140	7	18	2	2
Lowfat, baked	1 oz	115	1	22	2	4
Nacho flavor, regular	1 oz	140	7	18	2	2
Nacho flavor, reduced fat, baked	1 oz	125	4	20	1	2
(also see Corn Chips)	...	...	.	.	.	.
Tostada	...	...	.	.	.	.
Beef, bean, & cheese	1	330	17	30	2	16
Chicken & cheese	1	250	11	26	1	15
Guacamole	1	180	12	16	1	6
Trail Mix	...	...	.	.	.	.
Regular w/raisins, nuts, seeds,	...	...	.	.	.	.
& chocolate chips	1 cup	705	47	66	9	21
Tropical dried fruit mix	1 cup	570	24	92	11	9
Tuna – see Fish	...	...	.	.	.	.
Tuna Dishes	...	...	.	.	.	.
Tuna & broccoli w/creamy sauce	1 cup	300	12	31	1	14
Tuna & noodle casserole	1 cup	320	10	37	2	20
Tuna & pasta w/cheese sauce	1 cup	300	11	36	1	14
Tuna & pasta w/creamy sauce	1 cup	300	12	36	1	14
Tuna au gratin	1 cup	310	12	36	1	14
Tuna fettuccine alfredo	1 cup	310	14	32	1	14
Tuna romanoff	1 cup	280	8	38	1	15
Tuna tetrazzini	1 cup	310	12	33	1	17
Tuna Salad	...	...	.	.	.	.
Prep w/tuna in oil, regular	...	...	.	.	.	.

FOOD: (See Beverages & Fast Food Restaurants listed separately)	Serving Size	Cal- ories	Fat (g)	Carb (g)	Fi- ber (g)	Pro- tein (g)
mayo dressing, pickle relish	½ cup	190	10	9	0	16
Prep w/ tuna in water, light	...	...	.	.	.	.
mayo dressing, pickle relish	½ cup	130	5	6	0	15
TURKEY	...	...	.	.	.	.
Fried Turkey patty, battered	3 oz	250	15	14	Tr	12
Roast Turkey	...	...	.	.	.	.
light & dark meat	3 oz	145	5	3	0	22
light meat only	3 oz	135	4	0	0	25
dark meat only	3 oz	160	6	0	0	25
Giblets, simmered, chopped	1 cup	240	7	3	0	39
Ground Turkey	4 oz	195	11	0	0	22
Neck, simmered	2 slices	275	11	0	0	41
(Other Turkey Products, see:	...	...	.	.	.	.
Bologna, Hot Dog, Salami,	...	...	.	.	.	.
Sausage & specific entrées)	...	...	.	.	.	.
Turkey & Gravy	...	...	.	.	.	.
Banquet entrée	1 meal	140	9	6	Tr	8
Turkey Dijon	...	...	.	.	.	.
Lean Cuisine entrée	1 meal	280	10	21	1	26
Turkey Tetrazzini	...	...	.	.	.	.
Stouffers entrée	1 meal	360	17	33	1	19
Turmeric, ground	½ tsp	4	Tr	1	Tr	Tr
Turnip, sliced, cooked	½ cup	20	Tr	4	Tr	1
Turnip Greens, cooked	½ cup	16	Tr	3	Tr	1
Turnover	...	...	.	.	.	.
Apple or Cherry, large	1	410	16	63	4	4
Apple, small	1	170	8	21	2	2
Blueberry, small	1	165	8	23	2	2
Cherry, small	1	175	8	21	2	2
Vanilla Extract	1 tsp	12	Tr	1	0	Tr
Veal	...	...	.	.	.	.
Chop, loin, braised	3.5 oz	285	17	0	0	30
Cutlet, braised, lean & fat	3 oz	180	5	0	0	31
Liver, braised	3.5 oz	165	7	0	0	22
Rib, roasted, lean & fat	3.5 oz	250	13	0	0	24
Veal Marsala, Le Menu entrée	1 meal	250	5	25	1	25
Veal Parmagiana	.	.	.	.	.	.
Le Menu entrée	1 meal	175	6	9	Tr	22
Morton entrée	1 meal	280	13	30	1	8
Vegetable Burger, broiled	1 patty	100	1	9	4	15

FOOD: (See Beverages & Fast Food Restaurants listed separately)	Serving Size	Cal-ories	Fat (g)	Carb (g)	Fi-ber (g)	Pro-tein (g)
Vegetables, mixed	...	...	.	.	.	.
(See specific listings for	...	...	.	.	.	.
individual vegetables)	...	...	.	.	.	.
Mixed, canned, drained, heated	1 cup	80	Tr	15	5	4
Mixed, frozen, w/o sauce, heated	...	...	.	.	.	.
Small vegetables- peas, carrots,	...	...	.	.	.	.
beans, corn	1 cup	105	Tr	21	5	5
Large vegetable cuts- broccoli,	...	...	.	.	.	.
cauliflower, whole mushroom	1 cup	27	0	4	3	3
Large vegetable cuts	...	...	.	.	.	.
prep w/ butter sauce	1 cup	107	9	4	3	3
Vegetables, mixed, Birdseye	...	...	.	.	.	.
French style	¾ cup	110	2	10	3	6
Italian style	½ cup	100	6	11	3	2
Japanese style	½ cup	90	5	10	3	2
Mexican style	½ cup	140	5	24	3	5
Oriental style	½ cup	60	4	4	2	2
Vinegar	...	...	.	.	.	.
Regular	1 Tbsp	2	0	1	0	0
Cider vinegar	1 Tbsp	2	0	1	0	0
Waffle	...	...	.	.	.	.
Regular, prep from recipe, 7" dia	1 piece	215	11	25	1	6
Frozen, toaster size, 4 " dia	1 piece	90	3	13	1	2
Lowfat, toaster size, 4" dia	1 piece	80	1	15	Tr	2
Walnut – see Nuts	...	...	.	.	.	.
Water Chestnut, canned, slices	1 cup	75	Tr	17	4	1
Watercress, raw	½ cup	2	0	Tr	Tr	Tr
Watermelon	...	...	.	.	.	.
Fresh, diced	1 cup	50	1	11	1	1
Fresh, wedge, 1" thick, 1/16 of	...	...	.	.	.	.
melon 15" long x 7 ½" dia	1 wedge	92	1	21	1	2
Wheat Bran	¼ cup	25	1	3	1	2
Wheat Germ, toasted, plain	1 Tbsp	27	1	3	1	2
Whipped Cream – see Cream	...	...	.	.	.	.
Wiener – see Hot Dog	...	...	.	.	.	.
Yam – see Sweet Potato	...	...	.	.	.	.
Yeast	...	...	.	.	.	.
Compressed	1 cake	18	Tr	3	1	1
Dry, active, regular size pkg	1 pkg	21	Tr	3	2	3
Dry, active	1 tsp	12	Tr	2	1	2
Yogurt	...	...	.	.	.	.

FOOD: (See Beverages & Fast Food Restaurants listed separately)	Serving Size	Cal-ories	Fat (g)	Carb (g)	Fi-ber (g)	Pro-tein (g)
Chocolate, regular	½ cup	120	4	18	2	3
Chocolate, fat free	½ cup	90	0	17	1	5
Strawberry, regular	½ cup	120	4	19	Tr	4
Strawberry, fat free	½ cup	100	0	23	0	3
Vanilla, regular	½ cup	120	4	18	0	3
Vanilla, fat free	½ cup	110	0	23	0	4
Yogurt, plain,	...	...	.	.	.	.
made w/ whole milk	½ cup	140	7	11	0	8
made w/ lowfat milk	½ cup	130	3	19	0	11
made w/ skim milk	½ cup	120	0	15	0	13
Yogurt w/fruit, regular varieties	½ cup	135	3	20	1	5
Yogurt, w/fruit flavor, sugarfree	½ cup	95	Tr	16	0	9
Ziti w/ Meat Sauce	...	...	.	.	.	.
Swanson entrée	1 meal	560	23	58	1	28
Zucchini	...	...	.	.	.	.
Fresh, avg size	1	5	0	1	Tr	Tr
Sliced, cooked	½ cup	15	0	4	1	Tr
Breaded, fried	½ cup	165	9	16	2	4

FAST FOOD RESTAURANTS

FAST FOOD RESTAURANT: (See other Foods and Beverages listed separately)	Serving Size	Cal- ories	Fat (g)	Carb (g)	Fi- ber (g)	Pro- tein (g)
Arby's	...	...	.	.	.	.
Apple turnover	1	330	14	48	0	4
Arby-Q	1	430	18	48	3	22
Arby's melt w/ cheddar	1	370	18	36	2	18
Arby's sauce	1 svg	15	Tr	4	0	Tr
Bacon cheddar deluxe	1	540	34	38	3	22
Baked potato, deluxe	1	735	36	86	7	19
Baked potato, plain	1	355	Tr	82	7	7
Baked potato w/sour cream	1	580	24	85	7	9
Barbecue sauce	1 svg	30	0	7	0	0
Beef & cheddar sandwich	1	490	28	40	2	25
Beefstock Au Jus	1	10	0	1	0	0
Biscuit, plain	1	280	15	34	1	6
Bleu cheese dressing	1 svg	290	31	2	0	2
Blueberry muffin	1	230	9	35	0	2
Boston clam chowder	1 svg	190	9	18	1	9
Breaded chicken fillet	1	542	28	46	5	28
Broccoli & cheddar baked potato	1	580	20	89	9	14
Butterfinger polar swirl	1	455	18	62	0	15
Cheddar cheese sauce	1 svg	35	3	1	0	1
Cheddar curly fries	1 svg	335	18	40	3	3
Cheesecake, plain	1	320	23	23	1	5
Cherry turnover	1	320	13	46	1	4
Chicken Cordon Bleu	1	625	33	46	5	38
Chicken fingers, 2 pieces/svg	1 svg	290	16	20	1	16
Chocolate chip cookie	1	125	6	16	Tr	2
Chocolate shake	med	450	12	76	0	15
Cinnamon nut Danish	1	360	11	60	1	6
Cream of broccoli soup	1 svg	160	8	15	2	7
Croissant, plain	1	220	12	25	0	4
Curly fries	1 svg	300	15	38	0	4
Fish fillet	1	530	27	50	2	23
French dip	1 svg	475	22	40	3	30
French fries	1	240	13	30	3	2
French toast stix, 6 pieces/svg	1 svg	430	21	52	3	10
Garden salad w/o dressing	1	60	Tr	12	5	3

FAST FOOD RESTAURANT: (See other Foods and Beverages listed separately)	Serving Size	Cal-ories	Fat (g)	Carb (g)	Fi-ber (g)	Pro-tein (g)
Giant roast beef	1	555	28	43	5	35
Grilled chicken deluxe	1	430	20	41	3	23
Grilled chicken barbecue	1	390	13	47	2	23
Ham & cheese	1	355	14	24	2	24
Ham & cheese melt	1	335	13	34	2	20
Heath polar swirl	1	545	22	76	0	15
Honey French dressing	1 svg	275	23	18	0	0
Horsey sauce	1 svg	55	5	2	0	0
Hot ham & Swiss	1	500	23	43	2	30
Italian sub sandwich	1	670	36	46	2	30
Italian sub sauce	1 svg	70	7	1	0	0
Jamocha shake	small	385	10	62	0	15
Junior roast beef	1	325	14	35	2	17
Light mayonnaise	1 svg	12	1	1	Tr	0
Lumberjack mixed vegetables	1 svg	90	4	10	1	2
Old fashion chicken noodle soup	1 svg	80	2	11	1	6
Oreo polar swirl	1	480	22	66	1	15
Parmesan cheese sauce	1 svg	70	7	1	0	0
Peanut butter cup polar swirl	1	515	24	61	1	20
Philly beef & Swiss	1	750	47	48	3	39
Potato cakes	1 svg	200	12	20	2	2
Potato with bacon soup	1 svg	170	7	23	2	6
Red ranch dressing	1 svg	75	6	5	0	0
Reduced cal honey mayonnaise	1 svg	70	7	1	0	0
Reduced calorie Italian dressing	1 svg	20	1	3	0	0
Reduced cal buttermilk ranch	1 svg	50	Tr	12	0	0
Roast beef sandwich, regular	1	390	19	33	3	23
Roast beef deluxe sandwich	1	300	10	33	6	18
Roast beef sub sandwich	1	700	42	44	4	38
Roast chicken club	1	545	31	37	2	31
Roast chicken Santa Fe	1	435	22	35	1	29
Roast chicken deluxe	1	280	6	33	4	20
Roast chicken salad	1	150	2	12	5	20
Roast turkey deluxe	1	260	7	33	4	20
Side salad w/o dressing	1	25	Tr	4	2	1
Snickers polar swirl	1	510	19	73	1	15
Super roast beef	1	525	27	50	5	15
Tartar sauce	1 svg	140	15	0	0	0
Thousand island dressing	1 svg	260	26	7	0	0
Timberline chili	1 svg	220	10	17	7	18
Triple cheese melt	1	720	45	46	2	37

FAST FOOD RESTAURANT: (See other Foods and Beverages listed separately)	Serving Size	Cal- ories	Fat (g)	Carb (g)	Fi- ber (g)	Pro- tein (g)
Turkey sub sandwich	1	550	27	47	2	31
Upper ten	1	170	0	42	0	0
Vanilla shake	small	360	12	50	0	15
Wisconsin cheese soup	1 svg	280	18	20	2	10
Baskin Robbins	...	...	.	.	.	.
Aloha berry banana smoothie	1	165	Tr	36	1	3
Bora berry smoothie	1	175	Tr	38	2	4
Café mocha yogurt	1	80	Tr	15	1	4
Calypso berry smoothie	1	160	Tr	35	2	3
Chocolate chip ice cream	1	155	9	16	Tr	2
Chocolate chocolate chip, sugarfree	... 1	... 100	. 3	. 17	. Tr	. 4
Chocolate ice cream	1	155	8	19	Tr	3
Chocolate yogurt	1	80	0	15	1	5
Copa banana smoothie	1	145	Tr	30	1	4
Daiquiri ice	1	110	0	27	0	0
Dutch chocolate	1	105	Tr	23	1	4
Espresso & cream	1	110	4	18	0	3
Maui brownie madness	1	145	3	26	1	5
Perils of praline	1	130	3	24	0	4
Rainbow sherbet	1	120	2	25	0	1
Raspberry cheese Louise	1	135	3	24	0	4
Red raspberry sorbet	1	120	0	30	0	0
Rocky road ice cream	1	165	8	21	Tr	3
Silk chocolate	1	120	0	25	1	5
Strawberry yogurt, nonfat	1	105	0	23	0	3
Sunset orange smoothie	1	150	Tr	32	2	4
Thin mint, sugarfree	1	100	3	17	0	4
Tropic of fruit yogurt, nonfat	1	130	0	28	0	4
Tropical tango smoothie	1	180	Tr	40	1	4
Vanilla bean dream yogurt, nonfat	... 1	... 110	. 0	. 23	. 0	. 4
Vanilla bean dream	1	120	0	25	0	5
Vanilla chocolate twist, nonfat	1	100	0	21	1	4
Vanilla ice cream	1	145	8	14	0	3
Vanilla yogurt	1	80	0	15	1	4
Very berry strawberry ice cream	1	120	6	16	0	2

FAST FOOD RESTAURANT: (See other Foods and Beverages listed separately)	Serving Size	Cal- ories	Fat (g)	Carb (g)	Fi- ber (g)	Pro- tein (g)
Boston Market	…	…	.	.	.	.
Apples w/ cinnamon	1 svg	252	5	56	3	Tr
Barbecue baked beans	1 svg	330	9	53	9	11
Black beans with rice	1 svg	300	10	45	5	8
Broccoli and rice casserole	1svg	240	12	26	3	5
Brownie, chocolate	1	310	10	51	3	3
Cake, chocolate	1 piece	505	24	73	2	3
Cake, hummingbird	1 piece	705	36	92	2	6
Carrots, glazed	1 svg	280	15	35	2	1
Cheesecake	1 piece	575	41	44	1	9
Chicken with skin, ½	1	625	37	2	0	70
Chicken w/o skin, ¼, dark meat	1	210	10	1	0	28
Chicken with skin, ¼, dark meat	1	325	22	2	0	30
Chicken w/o skin, ¼, white meat	1	165	4	1	0	31
Chicken w/ skin, ¼, white meat	1	310	17	2	0	43
Chicken Caesar salad	1	670	47	16	2	45
Chicken pot pie	1	745	46	57	3	26
Chicken salad sandwich	1	675	30	63	3	39
Chicken sandwich	1	390	5	60	2	31
Chicken sandwich, barbecued	1	540	9	84	2	30
Chicken sandwich w/cheese	1	630	28	61	2	37
Cole slaw	1 svg	300	19	30	3	2
Cookie, chocolate chip	1	390	19	33	2	3
Cookie, oatmeal	1	390	20	47	2	5
Cookie, peanut butter	1	420	25	43	2	7
Corn, buttered w/herbs	1 svg	180	4	30	2	5
Corn, whole kernel	1 svg	180	4	30	2	5
Cornbread	1 svg	200	6	33	2	3
Cranberry relish	1 svg	330	5	70	2	1
Cranberry walnut relish	1 svg	365	6	75	3	3
Green beans	1 svg	80	6	5	3	1
Green bean casserole	1 svg	85	5	9	3	1
Ham with honey glaze	5 oz	210	8	10	1	24
Ham sandwich	1	410	8	65	2	25
Ham sandwich w/cheese & sauce	1	655	31	67	2	31
Macaroni and cheese	1 svg	280	11	33	3	13
Meatloaf	5 oz	290	17	15	1	20
Meatloaf sandwich w/ cheese	1	695	27	83	3	36
Meatloaf sandwich, open faced	1	730	36	74	2	29
Pie, apple streusel	1 piece	480	18	63	2	4
Pie, cherry streusel	1 piece	410	17	60	2	4

FAST FOOD RESTAURANT: (See other Foods and Beverages listed separately)	Serving Size	Cal- ories	Fat (g)	Carb (g)	Fi- ber (g)	Pro- tein (g)
Pie, pecan	1 piece	555	27	71	3	5
Pie, pumpkin	1 piece	370	17	50	2	5
Potatoes, dill & garlic	1 svg	130	3	25	2	3
Potatoes, mashed	1 svg	185	8	25	2	3
Potatoes, mashed w/gravy	1 svg	205	9	27	2	4
Potatoes, new	1 svg	130	3	25	2	3
Potato salad	1 svg	200	12	22	2	3
Red beans and rice	1 svg	260	5	45	3	8
Rice pilaf	1 svg	180	5	32	2	5
Salad, Caesar	1 svg	200	17	7	2	7
Salad, chunky chicken	1 svg	480	39	4	1	25
Salad, cucumber	1 svg	120	10	9	3	2
Salad, fruit	1 svg	70	1	15	3	1
Salad, tortellini	1 svg	350	24	24	3	11
Spinach, creamed	1 svg	260	20	11	3	9
Squash, butternut	1 svg	160	6	25	3	2
Squash casserole	1 svg	335	24	20	2	7
Stuffing, savory	1 svg	310	12	44	2	6
Sweet potato casserole	1 svg	280	18	39	3	3
Turkey bacon club sandwich	1	780	38	64	3	47
Turkey breast w/o skin	5 oz	170	1	1	0	36
Turkey sandwich, regular	1	390	4	61	2	33
Turkey sandwich w/cheese	1	615	25	64	2	39
Turkey sandwich, open faced	1	715	20	64	2	47
Vegetables, steamed, w/o sauce	1 svg	35	1	7	3	2
Zucchini marinara	1 svg	80	4	10	2	2
Burger King	...	...	.	.	.	.
A.M. express dip	1 svg	85	Tr	21	2	2
A.M. express grape jam	1 svg	30	0	7	Tr	0
A.M. express strawberry jam	1 svg	30	0	8	Tr	0
Bacon bits	1 svg	15	1	0	0	1
Barbecue sauce	1 svg	35	Tr	9	0	0
Barbecue sauce, bull's eye	1 svg	20	Tr	5	0	0
Biscuit with sausage	1	585	40	41	1	16
Biscuit w/ bacon, egg & cheese	1	510	31	39	1	19
BK big fish	1	695	41	56	3	26
BK broiler	1	550	29	41	2	30
Bleu cheese dressing	1 svg	160	16	1	0	2
Broiled chicken salad	1	200	10	7	3	21
Cheeseburger	1	385	19	28	1	23

FAST FOOD RESTAURANT: (See other Foods and Beverages listed separately)	Serving Size	Cal- ories	Fat (g)	Carb (g)	Fi- ber (g)	Pro- tein (g)
Chicken sandwich	1	705	43	54	2	26
Chicken tenders, 8 pieces/svg	1 svg	310	17	19	3	3
Chocolate shake	med	445	7	84	2	2
Croissanwich with sausage, egg & cheese	... 1	... 600	. 46	. 25	. 1	. 1
Croutons	1 svg	30	1	4	0	Tr
Double cheeseburger	1	605	36	28	1	1
Double cheeseburger w/ bacon	1	640	39	28	1	1
Double whopper	1	875	56	45	3	3
Double whopper w/ cheese	1	965	63	46	3	3
Dutch apple pie	1	300	15	39	2	2
French dressing	1 svg	145	10	11	0	Tr
French fries	med	375	20	43	3	3
French fries, coated	med	340	17	43	3	3
French toast sticks	1 svg	505	27	60	1	1
Garden salad w/o dressing	1	100	5	7	3	3
Hamburger	1	335	15	28	1	1
Hash browns	1	220	12	25	2	2
Honey dressing	1 svg	90	Tr	23	Tr	Tr
Land o'lakes classic whip blend	1 svg	65	7	0	0	0
Onion rings	1 svg	315	14	41	6	6
Ranch dressing	1 svg	175	17	2	0	0
Reduced calorie Italian dressing	1 svg	15	1	3	0	0
Side salad w/o dressing	1	60	3	4	2	2
Strawberry shake	med	425	6	93	1	1
Sweet & sour sauce	1 svg	45	0	11	0	0
Tartar sauce	1 svg	145	12	7	0	0
Thousand island dressing	1 svg	180	19	0	0	0
Vanilla shake	med	305	6	54	3	3
Whopper junior	1	425	24	29	2	2
Whopper junior w/ cheese	1	460	28	29	2	2
Whopper	1	645	38	45	3	3
Whopper w/ cheese	1	735	45	46	3	3
Chinese Restaurant – see Panda Express Chinese Food	... ...	... ...	. .	. .	. .	. .
Dairy Queen (all listings regular size, unless noted	... ...	... ...	. . .	. . .	. . .	. . .
Banana split	1	515	12	96	3	8
Buster bar	1	445	28	41	2	10

94

FAST FOOD RESTAURANT: (See other Foods and Beverages listed separately)	Serving Size	Cal-ories	Fat (g)	Carb (g)	Fi-ber (g)	Pro-tein (g)
Butterfinger blizzard	1	750	26	115	1	16
Caramel & nut bar	1	260	13	32	1	5
Chocolate cone	1	360	11	56	1	9
Chocolate soft serve	½ cup	150	5	22	1	4
Chocolate dilly bar	1	450	28	21	1	3
Chocolate dilly bar, mint	1	190	12	20	1	3
Chocolate malt	1	880	22	155	1	18
Chocolate shake	1	770	20	130	2	17
Chocolate sundae	1	410	10	73	1	8
Cookie dough blizzard	1	945	36	142	2	17
Dipped cone	1	515	25	63	1	9
DQ frozen heart cake	1 piece	270	9	41	2	5
DQ frozen log cake	1 piece	280	9	43	2	5
DQ frozen round cake	1 piece	340	12	53	2	7
DQ frozen sheet cake	1 piece	350	12	54	2	7
DQ fudge bar	1	60	Tr	13	Tr	3
DQ lemon freez'r	1	80	0	20	Tr	0
DQ orange bar	1	60	0	15	Tr	Tr
DQ sandwich	1	150	5	24	1	3
DQ vanilla orange bar	1	60	0	17	Tr	2
DQ vanilla soft serve	½ cup	140	5	22	Tr	3
DQ yogurt, nonfat frozen	½ cup	100	0	21	Tr	3
Fudge nut bar	1	410	25	40	2	8
Heath blizzard	1	818	33	119	2	14
Heath breeze	1	710	18	123	2	15
Heath treatzza pizza	1 slice	180	7	28	2	3
M&M treatzza pizza	1 slice	190	7	29	2	3
Misty slush	1	290	0	74	Tr	0
Oreo blizzard	1	640	23	79	2	10
Peanut buster parfait	1	730	31	99	2	16
Peanut butter fudge treatzza pizza	1 slice	220	10	28	2	4
Queen's choice choc. big scoop	1	250	14	28	2	4
Queen's choice vanilla big scoop	1	250	14	27	Tr	4
Reeses peanut butter cup blizzard	1	785	33	105	2	19
Starkiss	1	80	0	21	Tr	0
Strawberry banana treatzza pizza	1 slice	180	6	29	2	3
Strawberry blizzard	1	570	16	95	1	12
Strawberry breeze	1	460	1	99	1	13
Strawberry misty cooler	1	190	0	49	Tr	0
Strawberry shortcake	1 piece	430	14	24	2	7
Toffee dilly bar	1	210	12	24	1	3

FAST FOOD RESTAURANT: (See other Foods and Beverages listed separately)	Serving Size	Calories	Fat (g)	Carb (g)	Fiber (g)	Protein (g)
Vanilla cone	1	355	10	57	0	8
Vanilla cone, small	1	230	7	38	0	6
Yogurt cone	1	280	1	59	1	9
Yogurt cup	1	230	1	49	1	8
Yogurt strawberry sundae	1	305	1	66	1	10
Denny's	...	...	.	.	.	.
Banana split	1	885	43	121	3	15
Biscuit with sausage gravy	7 oz	395	21	45	2	8
Buffalo wings, 12 per svg	1 svg	855	54	1	Tr	92
Carrots with honey glaze	1 svg	80	3	12	2	1
Charleston chicken dinner	1	325	18	16	1	25
Cheesecake	1 slice	470	27	48	Tr	6
Cheese fries with chili	1 svg	815	44	77	3	29
Cheese fries, smothered	1 svg	765	48	69	3	27
Chicken burger sandwich	1	630	32	53	2	35
Chicken burger buffalo sandwich	1	800	45	67	2	37
Chicken fried steak	4 oz	265	17	14	1	15
Chicken strips, 5 per svg	1 svg	720	33	56	2	47
Chicken strips buffalo, 5 per svg	1 svg	735	42	43	1	48
Chili with cheese topping	1 svg	400	19	21	1	26
Chocolate layer cake	1 slice	275	12	42	2	4
Club sandwich	1	720	38	62	2	32
Corn with butter sauce	1 svg	120	4	19	2	3
Country fried potatoes	1 svg	515	35	23	3	3
Double scoop sundae	1	375	27	29	1	6
French fries	1 svg	260	12	35	3	5
French fries w/ seasoning	1 svg	320	14	44	4	5
Fried shrimp dinner	8 oz	220	10	18	1	17
Garden salad deluxe w/ chicken	1	265	11	10	5	32
Grasshopper blender blaster	15 oz	735	37	92	1	13
Grasshopper sundae	14 oz	735	34	97	1	13
Green beans w/ bacon	1 svg	60	4	6	2	1
Green peas w/ butter sauce	1 svg	100	2	14	3	5
Grilled chicken dinner	1	130	4	0	0	24
Grilled chicken sandwich	1	435	9	56	2	35
Grilled chicken stir fried	1	865	10	149	3	43
Grilled salmon dinner	6 oz	210	4	1	0	43
Ham & Swiss sandwich	1	535	31	40	2	23
Hamburger, bacon & cheddar	1	875	52	58	2	53
Hamburger, big Texas BBQ	1	930	58	53	2	53

FAST FOOD RESTAURANT: (See other Foods and Beverages listed separately)	Serving Size	Cal- ories	Fat (g)	Carb (g)	Fi- ber (g)	Pro- tein (g)
Hamburger, boca	1	615	28	66	2	29
Hamburger, classic	1	675	40	42	2	37
Hamburger, classic doubledecker	1	1375	92	81	3	62
Hamburger, classic w/ cheese	1	836	53	43	2	47
Hamburger, mushroom & Swiss	1	872	51	58	2	48
Hot fudge cake sundae	1 svg	620	35	73	2	7
Malted milk shake, chocolate	12 oz	585	26	82	1	12
Malted milk shake, vanilla	12 oz	585	26	82	Tr	12
Mashed potatoes	1 svg	105	1	21	2	3
Mashed potatoes w/ cheddar	1 svg	117	2	22	2	3
Mozzarella sticks, 8 per svg	1 svg	710	41	49	1	36
Onion rings	1 svg	380	23	38	2	5
Peaches and cream sundae	1	570	22	91	1	5
Pie, apple	1 slice	475	24	64	2	3
Pie, cherry	1 slice	630	25	101	3	3
Pie, chocolate peanut butter	1 slice	655	39	64	3	15
Pie, Hershey's chocolate chip	1 slice	600	36	58	2	6
Pie, Oreo cookies & cream	1 slice	650	40	67	2	6
Pot roast dinner	1	295	11	5	Tr	42
Roast turkey dinner	1	388	3	38	1	46
Rueben sandwich	1	580	35	37	2	27
Shake, chocolate	12 oz	560	26	76	1	11
Shake, vanilla	12 oz	560	26	76	Tr	11
Shrimp scampi skillet dinner	1 svg	290	19	3	Tr	25
Sirloin steak dinner	8 oz	340	28	1	0	18
Slim slam	12 oz	495	12	98	1	34
Steak and shrimp dinner	9 oz	640	42	31	1	36
Super bird sandwich	1	620	32	48	2	35
T-bone steak dinner	14 oz	860	65	0	0	65
Two egg breakfast	1	825	67	1	0	6
Turkey breast sandwich	1	475	26	39	2	23
Vegetable rice pilaf	1 svg	85	1	16	2	2
Western wings roundup	20 oz	1515	88	89	3	89
Domino's Pizza (1 slice= 1/8 pizza)	...	...	.	.	.	.
Feast Pizzas, Medium 12-inch	...	...	.	.	.	.
America's favorite	...	...	.	.	.	.
Classic hand-tossed	1 slice	255	12	29	2	10
Crunchy thin crust	1 slice	210	14	15	1	8
Ultimate deep dish	1 slice	310	17	29	2	12
Bacon cheeseburger	...	...	.	.	.	.

FAST FOOD RESTAURANT: (See other Foods and Beverages listed separately)	Serving Size	Cal- ories	Fat (g)	Carb (g)	Fi- ber (g)	Pro- tein (g)
Classic hand-tossed	1 slice	275	13	28	2	12
Crunchy thin crust	1 slice	225	15	14	1	10
Ultimate deep dish	1 slice	325	19	28	2	14
Barbecue	…	…	.	.	.	.
Classic hand-tossed	1 slice	250	10	31	1	11
Crunchy thin crust	1 slice	205	12	17	1	8
Ultimate deep dish	1 slice	304	15	32	2	12
Deluxe	…	…	.	.	.	.
Classic hand-tossed	1 slice	235	10	29	2	9
Crunchy thin crust	1 slice	185	12	15	1	7
Ultimate deep dish	1 slice	285	15	29	2	11
Extravaganzza	…	…	.	.	.	.
Classic hand-tossed	1 slice	290	14	30	2	13
Crunchy thin crust	1 slice	240	16	16	1	11
Ultimate deep dish	1 slice	340	20	30	2	14
Hawaiian	…	…	.	.	.	.
Classic hand-tossed	1 slice	225	8	30	2	10
Crunchy thin crust	1 slice	175	10	16	1	8
Ultimate deep dish	1 slice	275	13	30	2	12
Meatzza	…	…	.	.	.	.
Classic hand-tossed	1 slice	281	14	29	2	13
Crunchy thin crust	1 slice	232	15	15	1	11
Ultimate deep dish	1 slice	335	19	29	2	14
Pepperoni	…	…	.	.	.	.
Classic hand-tossed	1 slice	265	13	28	2	11
Crunchy thin crust	1 slice	215	14	14	1	9
Ultimate deep dish	1 slice	320	18	29	2	13
Veggie	…	…	.	.	.	.
Classic hand-tossed	1 slice	220	8	29	2	9
Crunchy thin crust	1 slice	170	10	15	1	7
Ultimate deep dish	1 slice	270	14	30	2	11
Feast Pizzas, Large 14-inch	…	…	.	.	.	.
America's favorite	…	…	.	.	.	.
Classic hand-tossed	1 slice	355	16	39	2	14
Crunchy thin crust	1 slice	285	19	20	2	11
Ultimate deep dish	1 slice	435	24	42	3	17
Bacon cheeseburger	…	…	.	.	.	.
Classic hand-tossed	1 slice	380	18	38	2	17
Crunchy thin crust	1 slice	310	21	19	1	14
Ultimate deep dish	1 slice	460	26	41	2	20
Barbecue	…	…	.	.	.	.

FAST FOOD RESTAURANT: (See other Foods and Beverages listed separately)	Serving Size	Cal- ories	Fat (g)	Carb (g)	Fi- ber (g)	Pro- tein (g)
Classic hand-tossed	1 slice	345	14	43	2	14
Crunchy thin crust	1 slice	275	16	24	1	11
Ultimate deep dish	1 slice	425	21	46	2	17
Deluxe	...	...	.	.	.	.
Classic hand-tossed	1 slice	315	13	39	2	13
Crunchy thin crust	1 slice	245	15	20	2	10
Ultimate deep dish	1 slice	395	20	42	3	15
Extravaganza	...	...	.	.	.	.
Classic hand-tossed	1 slice	388	19	40	3	17
Crunchy thin crust	1 slice	320	26	21	2	14
Ultimate deep dish	1 slice	470	19	43	3	20
Hawaiian	...	...	.	.	.	.
Classic hand-tossed	1 slice	310	11	41	2	14
Crunchy thin crust	1 slice	240	13	43	2	11
Ultimate deep dish	1 slice	390	18	21	3	17
Meatzza	...	...	.	.	.	.
Classic hand-tossed	1 slice	380	18	39	2	17
Crunchy thin crust	1 slice	310	20	20	2	14
Ultimate deep dish	1 slice	458	25	42	3	19
Pepperoni	...	...	.	.	.	.
Classic hand-tossed	1 slice	360	17	39	2	16
Crunchy thin crust	1 slice	295	19	20	1	13
Ultimate deep dish	1 slice	440	24	42	3	18
Veggie	...	...	.	.	.	.
Classic hand-tossed	1 slice	300	11	40	3	13
Crunchy thin crust	1 slice	230	14	43	2	10
Ultimate deep dish	1 slice	380	18	21	3	15
Medium 12-inch Pizzas	...	...	.	.	.	.
(regular, not Feast pizza)	...	...	.	.	.	.
Cheese	...	...	.	.	.	.
Classic hand-tossed	1 slice	185	6	28	1	7
Crunchy thin crust	1 slice	135	7	14	1	5
Ultimate deep dish	1 slice	240	11	28	2	9
Beef	...	...	.	.	.	.
Classic hand-tossed	1 slice	225	9	28	2	9
Crunchy thin crust	1 slice	175	11	14	1	7
Ultimate deep dish	1 slice	277	15	28	2	11
Green pepper, mushroom, onion	...	...	.	.	.	.
Classic hand-tossed	1 slice	190	6	29	2	8
Crunchy thin crust	1 slice	142	8	15	1	6
Ultimate deep dish	1 slice	244	11	30	2	9

FAST FOOD RESTAURANT: (See other Foods and Beverages listed separately)	Serving Size	Cal-ories	Fat (g)	Carb (g)	Fi-ber (g)	Pro-tein (g)
Ham	...	...	.	.	.	.
Classic hand-tossed	1 slice	195	6	28	1	9
Crunchy thin crust	1 slice	150	8	14	1	7
Ultimate deep dish	1 slice	250	12	28	2	11
Ham & pineapple	...	...	.	.	.	.
Classic hand-tossed	1 slice	200	6	29	2	9
Crunchy thin crust	1 slice	150	8	15	1	7
Ultimate deep dish	1 slice	250	12	30	2	10
Pepperoni	...	...	.	.	.	.
Classic hand-tossed	1 slice	223	9	28	2	9
Crunchy thin crust	1 slice	175	11	14	1	7
Ultimate deep dish	1 slice	275	14	28	2	11
Pepperoni & sausage	...	...	.	.	.	.
Classic hand-tossed	1 slice	255	12	28	2	10
Crunchy thin crust	1 slice	206	14	14	1	8
Ultimate deep dish	1 slice	307	17	29	2	12
Sausage	...	...	.	.	.	.
Classic hand-tossed	1 slice	230	10	28	2	9
Crunchy thin crust	1 slice	181	11	14	1	7
Ultimate deep dish	1 slice	283	15	29	2	11
Large 14-inch Pizzas	...	...	.	.	.	.
(regular, not Feast pizza)	...	...	.	.	.	.
Cheese	...	...	.	.	.	.
Classic hand-tossed	1 slice	256	8	38	2	10
Crunchy thin crust	1 slice	190	10	19	1	7
Ultimate deep dish	1 slice	336	15	41	2	13
Beef	...	...	.	.	.	.
Classic hand-tossed	1 slice	310	13	38	2	13
Crunchy thin crust	1 slice	243	15	19	1	10
Ultimate deep dish	1 slice	390	20	41	2	15
Green pepper, mushroom, onion	...	...	.	.	.	.
Classic hand-tossed	1 slice	263	8	39	2	11
Crunchy thin crust	1 slice	200	10	21	2	8
Ultimate deep dish	1 slice	343	15	42	3	13
Ham	...	...	.	.	.	.
Classic hand-tossed	1 slice	270	9	38	2	12
Crunchy thin crust	1 slice	204	11	19	1	9
Ultimate deep dish	1 slice	350	16	41	2	15
Ham & pineapple	...	...	.	.	.	.
Classic hand-tossed	1 slice	275	9	40	2	12
Crunchy thin crust	1 slice	207	11	21	1	9

FAST FOOD RESTAURANT: (See other Foods and Beverages listed separately)	Serving Size	Cal-ories	Fat (g)	Carb (g)	Fi-ber (g)	Pro-tein (g)
Ultimate deep dish Pepperoni	1 slice	355	16	42	2	14
...	...	...	.	.	.	.
Classic hand-tossed	1 slice	305	12	38	2	12
Crunchy thin crust	1 slice	237	15	19	1	10
Ultimate deep dish Pepperoni & sausage	1 slice	385	20	41	2	15
...	...	...	.	.	.	.
Classic hand-tossed	1 slice	350	16	39	2	14
Crunchy thin crust	1 slice	282	19	19	2	11
Ultimate deep dish Sausage	1 slice	430	23	41	3	17
...	...	...	.	.	.	.
Classic hand-tossed	1 slice	320	14	39	2	13
Crunchy thin crust	1 slice	250	16	20	2	10
Ultimate deep dish	1 slice	400	21	42	3	15
Side Orders & Condiments	...	...	.	.	.	.
Barbecue buffalo wings	1 piece	50	3	2	0	6
Blue cheese dipping sauce	1 svg	225	24	2	0	1
Bread sticks	1 piece	115	6	12	0	2
Buffalo chicken kickers	1 piece	47	2	3	0	4
Cheesy bread	1 piece	125	7	13	0	4
Cinnamon stix	1 piece	125	6	15	1	2
Garlic sauce	1 svg	440	49	0	0	0
Hot buffalo wings	1 piece	45	3	1	0	5
Hot dipping sauce	1 svg	15	0	4	0	0
Marinara dipping sauce	1 svg	25	Tr	5	0	1
Ranch dipping sauce	1 svg	195	21	2	0	1
Sweet icing	1 svg	250	3	57	0	0
Dunkin' Donuts	...	...	.	.	.	.
Bagels	...	...	.	...	...	.
Berry berry	1	345	3	69	4	11
Blueberry	1	350	3	69	4	11
Cinnamon raisin	1	335	3	65	3	10
Everything	1	430	7	75	3	17
Garlic	1	410	4	79	3	16
Onion	1	375	4	71	4	14
Plain	1	360	3	69	2	14
Poppyseed	1	440	10	72	3	17
Salt	1	360	3	69	2	14
Sesame	1	455	11	71	3	18
Sourdough	1	340	3	65	2	15
Wheat	1	350	5	66	4	13

FAST FOOD RESTAURANT: (See other Foods and Beverages listed separately)	Serving Size	Cal- ories	Fat (g)	Carb (g)	Fi- ber (g)	Pro- tein (g)
Cream cheese	...	...	.	...	.	.
Chive	2 oz	170	17	4	2	4
Garden vegetable	2 oz	170	15	4	0	2
Light	2 oz	110	9	6	0	4
Plain	2 oz	190	17	4	0	4
Salmon	2 oz	170	17	2	0	4
Shedd's buttermatch blend	1 Tbsp	80	9	0	0	0
Strawberry	2 oz	195	17	9	0	4
Cookies	...	...	.	...	.	.
Chocolate chunk	1	220	11	28	1	3
Chocolate chunk w/ walnuts	1	230	12	27	1	3
Oatmeal raisin pecan	1	220	10	29	1	3
White chocolate chunk	1	235	12	28	1	3
Danish	...	...	.	...	.	.
Apple	1	250	10	36	0	4
Cheese	1	275	14	32	0	4
Strawberry cheese	1	250	12	33	0	4
Donuts	...	...	.	...	.	.
Apple crumb	1	235	10	34	1	3
Apple & spice	1	200	8	29	1	3
Bavarian kreme	1	210	9	30	1	3
Black raspberry	1	210	8	32	1	3
Blueberry cake	1	290	16	35	1	3
Blueberry crumb	1	240	10	36	1	3
Boston kreme	1	240	9	36	1	3
Chocolate coconut cake	1	300	19	31	1	4
Chocolate frosted cake	1	360	20	40	1	4
Chocolate frosted	1	200	9	29	1	3
Chocolate glazed cake	1	295	16	33	1	3
Chocolate kreme filled	1	270	13	35	1	3
Cinnamon cake	1	330	20	34	1	4
Double chocolate cake	1	310	17	39	2	3
French cruller	1	150	18	17	1	2
Glazed cake	1	350	19	41	1	4
Glazed	1	180	8	25	1	3
Jelly filled	1	210	8	32	1	3
Maple frosted	1	210	9	30	1	3
Marble frosted	1	200	9	29	1	3
Old fashioned cake	1	300	19	28	1	4
Powdered cake	1	330	19	36	1	4
Strawberry	1	210	8	32	1	3

FAST FOOD RESTAURANT: (See other Foods and Beverages listed separately)	Serving Size	Cal- ories	Fat (g)	Carb (g)	Fi- ber (g)	Pro- tein (g)
Strawberry frosted	1	210	9	30	1	3
Sugar raised	1	170	8	22	1	3
Vanilla kreme filled	1	170	13	36	1	3
Whole white glazed cake	1	310	19	32	1	4
Donut-Fancies	...	...	.	.	.	.
Apple fritter	1	300	14	41	1	4
Bow tie donut	1	300	17	34	1	4
Chocolate frosted coffee roll	1	290	15	36	1	4
Chocolate iced Bismarck	1	340	15	50	1	3
Coffee roll	1	270	14	33	1	4
Éclair	1	270	11	39	1	3
Glazed fritter	1	260	14	31	1	4
Maple frosted coffee roll	1	290	14	36	1	4
Vanilla frosted coffee roll	1	290	14	36	1	4
Donut-Munchkins	...	...	.	.	.	.
Cinnamon cake	4	275	15	31	1	3
Glazed	5	200	9	27	1	3
Glazed cake	3	280	13	38	1	3
Glazed chocolate cake	3	200	10	26	1	2
Jelly filled	5	210	9	30	1	3
Lemon filled	4	170	8	23	0	2
Plain cake	4	270	16	27	1	3
Powdered cake	4	270	14	31	1	3
Sugar raised	7	220	12	26	1	4
Donut-Sticks	...	...	.	.	.	.
Cinnamon cake	1	450	30	42	1	4
Glazed cake	1	490	29	51	1	4
Glazed chocolate cake	1	470	29	49	2	4
Jelly	1	530	29	61	1	4
Plain cake	1	420	29	35	1	4
Powdered cake	1	450	29	42	1	4
Muffins	...	...	.	.	.	.
Banana walnut	1	545	23	73	3	10
Blueberry	1	490	18	75	2	8
Carrot walnut spice	1	600	27	81	3	8
Chocolate chip	1	590	23	85	3	9
Coffee cake with topping	1	710	29	102	2	11
Corn	1	510	17	81	1	9
Cranberry orange	1	460	16	71	3	8
Honey bran raisin	1	490	14	81	5	10
Reduced fat blueberry	1	450	13	74	2	9

FAST FOOD RESTAURANT: (See other Foods and Beverages listed separately)	Serving Size	Cal- ories	Fat (g)	Carb (g)	Fi- ber (g)	Pro- tein (g)
Other Misc. Items	...	...	.	...	.	.
Apple pie	1 svg	615	28	82	4	9
Apple pie a la mode	1 svg	810	38	107	4	12
Biscuit, plain	1	250	13	29	1	5
Croissant, plain	1	330	18	37	0	5
Scone, maple walnut	1	470	22	62	1	6
Scone, raspberry white choc.	1	450	22	59	2	6
Sandwiches, Breakfast type	...	...	.	.	.	.
Bagel w/ egg, bacon, cheese	1	500	13	71	2	26
Bagel w/ egg, ham, cheese	1	500	11	70	2	29
Bagel w/ egg, sausage, cheese	1	675	28	71	2	32
Biscuit w/ egg & cheese	1	360	20	31	1	14
Biscuit w/ sausage, egg, cheese	1	560	38	31	1	23
Croissant w/ egg, ham, cheese	1	470	27	38	0	20
English muffin w/egg, cheese	1	270	8	35	1	15
English muffin w/ egg, bacon & cheese	... 1	... 310	. 11	. 35	. 1	. 18
English muffin w/ egg, ham, & cheese	... 1	... 310	. 10	. 35	. 1	. 21
Beverages	...	...	.	.	.	.
Cappuccino	10 oz	80	5	7	0	4
Cappuccino with sugar	10 oz	130	5	21	0	4
Coffee	10 oz	15	0	3	0	1
Coffee with cream	10 oz	70	6	3	0	1
Coffee with cream and sugar	10 oz	120	6	15	0	1
Coffee with milk	10 oz	35	1	4	0	2
Coffee with milk and sugar	10 oz	80	1	16	0	2
Coffee with skim milk	10 oz	25	0	4	0	2
Coffee w/ skim milk and sugar	10 oz	70	0	16	0	2
Coffee with sugar	10 oz	60	0	15	0	1
Coffee coolatta with 2% milk	16 oz	190	2	41	0	4
Coffee coolatta with cream	16 oz	350	22	40	0	3
Coffee coolatta with milk	16 oz	210	4	42	0	4
Coffee coolatta with skim milk	16 oz	170	0	41	0	4
Coolatta, lemonade	16 oz	240	0	59	0	0
Coolatta, orange mango	16 oz	270	0	66	2	1
Coolatta, strawberry fruit	16 oz	290	0	72	1	0
Coolatta, vanilla bean	16 oz	440	17	70	1	1
Dunkaccino	10 oz	230	10	35	0	2
Espresso	2 oz	1	0	1	0	0
Espresso with sugar	2 oz	30	0	7	0	0

FAST FOOD RESTAURANT: (See other Foods and Beverages listed separately)	Serving Size	Cal-ories	Fat (g)	Carb (g)	Fi-ber (g)	Pro-tein (g)
Hot chocolate	10 oz	220	8	38	2	2
Latte, plain	10 oz	120	6	10	0	6
Latte with sugar	10 oz	160	6	22	0	6
Latte w/ Caramel swirl	10 oz	230	6	36	0	8
Latte w/ Mocha swirl	10 oz	230	7	37	1	6
Iced coffee	16 oz	15	0	3	0	1
Iced coffee with cream	16 oz	70	6	4	0	2
Iced coffee w/ cream and sugar	16 oz	120	6	16	0	2
Iced coffee with milk	16 oz	35	1	4	0	2
Iced coffee w/ milk and sugar	16 oz	80	1	16	0	2
Iced coffee with skim milk	16 oz	25	0	4	0	2
Iced coffee w/skim milk, sugar	16 oz	70	0	16	0	2
Iced coffee with sugar	16 oz	60	0	15	0	1
Iced latte	16 oz	120	7	11	0	6
Iced latte with sugar	16 oz	170	7	23	0	6
Iced caramel swirl latte	16 oz	240	7	37	0	8
Iced mocha swirl latte	16 oz	240	8	38	1	7
Vanilla chai	10 oz	230	8	40	0	1
Tea, plain, w/o milk or sugar	...	...	.	.	.	.
Decaffeinated tea	10 oz	0	0	1	0	0
Earl Grey tea	10 oz	0	0	1	0	0
English breakfast tea	10 oz	0	0	1	0	0
Green tea	10 oz	0	0	1	0	0
Regular tea	10 oz	0	0	1	0	0
Regular tea w/ lemon	10 oz	0	0	1	0	0
Tea w/ regular milk, no sugar	10 oz	25	1	2	0	1
Tea w/ regular milk and sugar	10 oz	70	1	14	0	1
Tea w/ skim milk, no sugar	10 oz	25	Tr	4	0	1
Tea w/ skim milk and sugar	10 oz	60	Tr	14	0	1
Hardees	...	...	.	.	.	.
Apple cinnamon raisin biscuit	1	200	8	30	2	2
Bacon & egg biscuit	1	575	33	45	2	22
Bacon, egg & cheese biscuit	1	610	37	45	2	24
Baked beans	1 svg	170	1	32	4	8
Big chocolate chip cookie	1	280	12	41	2	4
Big country bacon	1 svg	820	49	62	2	33
Big country sausage	1 svg	995	66	62	2	41
Big roast beef	1	465	24	35	3	26
Biscuits w/ gravy	1 svg	495	28	55	3	10
Cheeseburger	1	310	14	30	2	16

FAST FOOD RESTAURANT: (See other Foods and Beverages listed separately)	Serving Size	Cal- ories	Fat (g)	Carb (g)	Fi- ber (g)	Pro- tein (g)
Chicken, breast	1 piece	370	15	29	2	29
Chicken, leg	1 piece	170	7	15	1	13
Chicken, thigh	1 piece	330	15	30	2	39
Chicken, wing	1 piece	195	8	23	1	10
Chicken fillet sandwich	1	480	18	54	3	26
Chocolate cone	1	180	3	34	1	5
Chocolate shake	1	375	5	67	1	13
Cole slaw	1 svg	240	20	13	3	2
Cool twist cone	1	180	2	34	1	4
Country ham biscuit	1	430	22	45	3	15
Cravin bacon cheeseburger	1	690	46	38	2	30
Fat free French dressing	1 svg	70	0	17	Tr	0
Fisherman's fillet	1	565	27	54	3	26
French fries, large	1	430	18	59	4	6
French fries, medium	1	350	15	49	3	5
French fries, small	1	240	10	33	2	4
Frisco ham sandwich	1	500	25	46	3	24
Frisco sandwich	1	720	46	43	3	33
Garden salad	1	220	13	11	3	12
Gravy, 1.5 oz	1 svg	22	1	3	Tr	1
Grilled chicken	1	350	11	38	2	25
Chilled chicken salad	1	150	3	11	3	20
Ham biscuit	1	400	30	47	3	9
Ham, egg, & cheese biscuit	1	540	30	48	3	20
Hamburger	1	270	11	29	2	14
Hot fudge sundae	1	180	6	51	1	7
Hot ham & cheese	1	310	12	34	2	16
Jelly biscuit	1	440	21	57	3	6
Mashed potatoes	1 svg	70	1	14	3	2
Mesquite bacon cheeseburger	1	370	18	32	2	19
Mushroom & Swiss burger	1	490	25	39	2	28
Pancakes, 3 per svg	1 svg	280	2	56	3	8
Peach cobbler	1 svg	310	7	60	2	2
Peach shake	1	390	4	77	1	10
Quarter Lb double cheeseburger	1	470	27	31	3	27
Ranch dressing	1 svg	290	29	6	Tr	1
Regular hash rounds	1 svg	230	14	24	2	3
Regular roast beef	1	320	16	26	2	17
Rise & shine biscuit	1	390	21	44	2	6
Sausage biscuit	1	510	31	44	2	14
Sausage & egg biscuit	1	630	40	45	2	23

FAST FOOD RESTAURANT: (See other Foods and Beverages listed separately)	Serving Size	Cal- ories	Fat (g)	Carb (g)	Fi- ber (g)	Pro- tein (g)
Side salad, w/o dressing	1	25	Tr	4	2	1
Strawberry shake	1	420	4	83	1	11
Strawberry sundae	1	210	2	43	1	5
The boss	1	570	33	42	3	27
The works burger	1	530	30	41	3	25
Thousand island dressing	1 svg	250	23	9	Tr	1
Ultimate omelet biscuit	1	570	33	45	2	22
Vanilla cone	1	170	2	34	1	4
Vanilla shake	1	350	5	65	1	12
Jack-In-The-Box	...	...	.	.	.	.
Breakfast Jack	1	295	12	30	1	18
Breakfast sandwich, sourdough	1	380	20	31	2	21
Carrot cake	1 piece	365	15	58	2	3
Cheeseburger, regular	1	320	15	32	2	16
Cheeseburger, double	1	450	24	35	2	24
Cheeseburger, ultimate	1	1025	79	30	3	50
Cheesecake	1 piece	310	18	29	1	8
Chicken pita fajita	1	290	8	29	2	24
Chicken sandwich, regular	1	400	18	38	2	20
Chicken sandwich, Caesar	1	520	26	44	2	27
Chicken sandwich, grilled	1	430	19	36	2	29
Chicken sandwich, spicy	1	560	27	55	2	24
Chicken sandwich, super	1	615	36	48	2	25
Chicken strips, 6 per svg	1 svg	450	20	28	1	39
Chicken teriyaki	1 svg	580	2	115	5	28
Egg roll	1 piece	150	8	18	1	1
Egg rolls, 5 piece serving	5 piece	745	41	92	3	5
French fries, curly	1	360	20	39	3	5
French fries, jumbo size	1	400	19	51	3	5
French fries, regular size	1	350	17	45	3	4
French fries, small	1	220	11	28	2	3
French fries, super size	1	590	29	76	5	8
Hamburger	1	280	11	31	2	13
Hash browns	2 oz	160	11	14	2	1
Jalapenos, stuffed	1 svg	600	39	41	2	22
Jumbo Jack	1	560	32	41	2	26
Jumbo Jack w/ cheese	1	650	40	42	2	31
Onion rings	1 svg	380	23	38	2	5
Pancake platter	1 svg	400	12	59	3	13
Potato wedges, bacon & cheddar	1 svg	795	58	49	4	20

FAST FOOD RESTAURANT: (See other Foods and Beverages listed separately)	Serving Size	Cal- ories	Fat (g)	Carb (g)	Fi- ber (g)	Pro- tein (g)
Sausage croissant	1	675	48	39	2	21
Scrambled egg pocket	1	430	21	31	1	29
Shake, cappuccino	1 large	625	28	80	1	11
Shake, chocolate	1 large	625	27	85	1	11
Shake, strawberry	1 large	630	28	85	1	10
Shake, vanilla	1 large	615	30	73	0	12
Supreme croissant	1	570	36	39	2	21
Taco	1	185	11	15	2	7
Taco monster	1	285	17	22	3	12
Kentucky Fried Chicken	…	…	.	.	.	.
Barbecue baked beans	1 svg	185	3	33	6	6
Biscuit	1	180	10	20	2	4
Breast, extra tasty crispy	1	470	28	25	1	31
Breast, hot & spicy	1	520	34	23	1	32
Breast, original recipe	1	400	25	16	1	29
Breast, tender roast	1	255	24	1	Tr	29
Chunky chicken pot pie	1	775	42	69	4	29
Coleslaw	5 oz	180	9	21	4	2
Cornbread	1 piece	228	13	18	3	27
Corn on the cob	1	190	3	34	4	5
Crispy strips, 3 pieces/svg	1 svg	260	16	10	3	20
Drumstick, original recipe	1	160	9	6	1	15
Drumstick, tender roast	1	100	4	1	0	13
Green beans	1 svg	45	5	7	3	1
Hot wings, 6 pieces/svg	1 svg	470	33	18	2	27
Kentucky nuggets , 6 pieces/svg	1 svg	285	18	15	1	16
Macaroni and cheese	med	180	8	21	3	7
Original recipe chicken	…	…	.	.	.	.
sandwich	1	495	22	46	3	29
Potato salad	1 svg	230	14	23	3	4
Potato wedges	1 svg	280	13	28	3	5
Potatoes, mashed	1 svg	120	6	17	3	1
Red beans and rice	1 svg	130	3	21	3	5
Thigh, extra tasty crispy or hot	1	370	25	18	1	19
Thigh, original recipe	1	255	18	6	1	16
Thigh, tender roast	1	205	12	1	0	18
Value BBQ chicken sandwich	1	255	8	28	2	17
Wing, extra tasty crispy or hot	1	210	15	9	1	10
Wing, original recipe	1	140	10	5	Tr	9
Wing, tender roast	1	121	8	1	Tr	12

FAST FOOD RESTAURANT: (See other Foods and Beverages listed separately)	Serving Size	Cal- ories	Fat (g)	Carb (g)	Fi- ber (g)	Pro- tein (g)
Krispy Kreme Doughnuts	...	...	.	.	.	.
Apple fritter	1	385	21	46	Tr	4
Caramel creme crunch	1	350	19	43	Tr	4
Chocolate iced cake	1	270	14	36	Tr	3
Chocolate iced cake w/ sprinkles	1	290	14	40	Tr	3
Chocolate iced crème filled	1	350	21	39	Tr	3
Chocolate iced cruller	1	290	15	37	Tr	2
Chocolate iced custard filled	1	300	17	35	Tr	3
Chocolate iced glazed	1	250	12	33	Tr	3
Chocolate iced glazed, sprinkles	1	200	12	38	Tr	3
Chocolate malted kreme	1	395	21	49	Tr	4
Cinnamon apple filled	1	290	16	32	Tr	3
Cinnamon bun	1	260	16	28	Tr	3
Cinnamon sugar cake	1	280	14	37	Tr	3
Cinnamon twist	1	230	9	33	Tr	3
Coffee & kreme	1	360	20	43	Tr	3
Dulce de leche	1	295	18	30	Tr	3
Glazed blueberry cake	1	340	18	42	Tr	3
Glazed blueberry filled	1	290	16	35	Tr	3
Glazed cinnamon	1	210	12	24	Tr	2
Glazed crème filled	1	345	20	39	Tr	3
Glazed cruller	1	240	14	26	Tr	2
Glazed custard filled	1	290	16	34	Tr	3
Glazed devil's food cake	1	340	18	42	Tr	3
Glazed lemon filled	1	290	16	34	Tr	3
Glazed sour cream	1	340	18	42	Tr	3
Glazed raspberry filled	1	300	16	39	Tr	3
Glazed strawberry filled	1	290	16	35	Tr	3
Glazed twist	1	210	9	28	Tr	3
Honey and oat	1	340	18	42	Tr	3
Key lime pie	1	330	18	40	Tr	3
Maple iced	1	240	12	32	Tr	2
Maple iced cake	1	270	13	35	Tr	3
New York cheesecake	1	330	19	36	Tr	4
Original glazed	1	200	12	22	Tr	2
Powdered blueberry filled	1	290	16	32	Tr	3
Powdered cake	1	280	14	37	Tr	3
Powdered crème filled	1	345	21	36	Tr	3
Powdered raspberry	1	300	16	36	Tr	3
Powdered strawberry filled	1	260	16	26	Tr	3

FAST FOOD RESTAURANT: (See other Foods and Beverages listed separately)	Serving Size	Cal- ories	Fat (g)	Carb (g)	Fi- ber (g)	Pro- tein (g)
Pumpkin spice cake	1	340	18	42	Tr	3
Sugar coated	1	200	12	21	Tr	2
Traditional cake	1	230	13	25	Tr	3
Vanilla iced cake w/ sprinkles	1	270	13	35	Tr	3
Vanilla iced crème filled	1	345	20	38	Tr	3
Vanilla iced custard filled	1	290	16	33	Tr	3
Vanilla iced glazed	1	240	12	32	Tr	2
Vanilla iced raspberry filled	1	355	16	50	Tr	3
Vanilla iced raspberry glazed	1	355	16	50	Tr	3
Long John Silver's	...	.	.	.	.	.
Cheesesticks, 3 per svg	1 svg	165	9	12	1	6
Chicken, battered plank	1	145	8	9	1	8
Chicken sandwich	1	340	14	40	2	13
Chicken sandwich w/ cheese	1	390	19	40	2	16
Clam chowder	1 svg	525	24	52	4	24
Clams, breaded	1 svg	250	14	26	2	9
Cole slaw	4 oz	170	7	23	5	2
Crabcake	1	150	9	12	1	4
Fish, battered	1 piece	230	13	16	2	12
Fish, battered, junior size	1 piece	120	8	8	1	5
Fish, country breaded	1 piece	200	10	17	2	10
Fish w/lemon crumb	2 piece	240	12	10	2	23
Fish sandwich	1	430	20	46	3	16
Fish sandwich w/ cheese	1	485	25	46	3	19
Fish sandwich, ultimate	1	490	26	46	3	19
French fries, regular size	1	250	15	28	2	3
French fries, large size	1	420	24	46	4	5
Grilled chicken salad	1	140	3	20	3	10
Hushpuppies	2 piece	120	6	50	2	18
Ocean chef salad	1	128	2	15	3	14
Pie, banana split sundae	1 svg	300	17	34	2	4
Pie, chocolate crème	1 svg	285	17	29	3	4
Pie, Dutch apple	1 svg	290	13	44	3	2
Pie, pecan	1 svg	390	19	53	3	3
Pie, strawberries & cream	1 svg	280	15	32	3	4
Pineapple crème cheesecake	1 svg	310	17	36	3	4
Shrimp, battered	1 piece	45	3	3	1	2
Shrimp, battered, popcorn	1 svg	325	15	33	3	15

FAST FOOD RESTAURANT: (See other Foods and Beverages listed separately)	Serving Size	Cal- ories	Fat (g)	Carb (g)	Fi- ber (g)	Pro- tein (g)
McDonald's	...	...	.	.	.	.
Apple bran muffin, lowfat	1	300	3	61	3	6
Apple Danish	1	360	16	51	1	5
Apple pie, baked	1	260	13	34	1	3
Arch deluxe	1	550	31	69	4	28
Arch deluxe with bacon	1	590	34	38	4	32
Bacon, egg & cheese biscuit	1	440	26	33	1	17
Barbecue sauce	1 svg	45	0	10	0	0
Big mac	1	560	31	45	3	26
Biscuit, plain	1	260	13	32	1	4
Breakfast burrito	1	320	20	23	1	13
Caesar salad	1	160	14	7	0	2
Chef salad	1	230	13	8	3	21
Cheese Danish	1	410	22	47	0	7
Cheeseburger	1	320	13	35	2	15
Chicken McNuggets, 4 pieces	1 svg	190	11	10	0	12
Chicken McNuggets, 6 pieces	1 svg	290	17	15	0	18
Chicken McNuggets, 9 pieces	1 svg	430	26	23	0	27
Chocolate chip cookie	1	170	10	22	1	2
Chocolate shake, small	1	360	9	60	1	11
Cinnamon roll	1	400	20	47	2	7
Crispy chicken deluxe	1	500	25	43	3	26
Croutons	1 svg	50	5	7	0	2
Egg McMuffin	1	290	12	27	1	17
English muffin	1	140	2	25	1	4
Fat free herb vinegar dressing	1 svg	50	0	11	0	1
Fish fillet sandwich	1	560	28	54	4	23
French fries, large	1	450	22	57	5	6
French fries, small	1	210	10	26	2	3
Garden salad	1	35	0	7	2	2
Grilled chicken deluxe	1	440	20	38	3	27
Grilled chicken salad deluxe	1	120	2	7	2	21
Hamburger	1	260	9	34	2	13
Hash browns	1 svg	130	7	53	2	9
Honey dressing	1 svg	45	0	12	0	0
Honey mustard dressing	1 svg	50	5	3	0	0
Hot caramel sundae	1	360	10	61	0	7
Hot fudge sundae	1	340	12	52	1	8
Hot mustard	1 svg	60	4	7	0	1
Hotcakes, plain	1 svg	310	7	53	2	9
Hotcakes w/ syrup & margarine	1 svg	580	16	100	2	9

111

FAST FOOD RESTAURANT: (See other Foods and Beverages listed separately)	Serving Size	Cal- ories	Fat (g)	Carb (g)	Fi- ber (g)	Pro- tein (g)
Mayonnaise, light	1 svg	40	4	0	0	0
McDonaldland cookie	1	180	5	32	1	3
Quarter pounder	1	420	21	37	2	23
Quarter pounder with cheese	1	530	30	38	2	28
Red French reduced cal dressing	1 svg	160	8	23	0	0
Sausage (w/o biscuit)	1 svg	170	16	0	0	6
Sausage biscuit w/ egg	1	505	35	33	1	16
Sausage McMuffin	1	360	23	26	1	13
Sausage McMuffin with egg	1	440	28	27	1	19
Scrambled eggs, 2 per svg	1 svg	160	11	1	0	13
Strawberry shake, small	1	360	9	60	0	11
Strawberry sundae	1	290	7	50	0	7
Sweet & sour sauce	1 svg	50	0	11	0	0
Vanilla cone, reduced fat	1	150	5	23	0	4
Vanilla shake, small	1	360	9	59	0	11
Panda Express Chinese Food	...	...	.	.	.	.
Beef dishes	...	...	.	.	.	.
Beef with broccoli	6 oz	150	8	8	1	11
Beef with string beans	6 oz	170	9	11	2	12
Chicken dishes	...	...	.	.	.	.
Black pepper chicken	6 oz	180	10	10	2	13
Chicken & orange sauce	6 oz	480	21	50	2	21
Chicken with mushrooms	6 oz	130	7	7	2	11
Chicken with string beans	6 oz	170	8	12	3	11
Hot spicy chicken w/ peanuts	6 oz	200	7	17	4	18
Mandarin chicken	6 oz	250	9	8	2	34
Potatoes with chicken	6 oz	220	11	17	1	12
Sweet & sour chicken	4 oz	310	14	28	2	18
Pork dishes	...	...	.	.	.	.
Barbecue pork	5 oz	350	19	13	Tr	32
Sweet & sour pork	4 oz	410	30	17	3	19
Vegetable dishes	...	...	.	.	.	.
Mixed vegetables	6 oz	70	3	8	3	3
String beans w/fried tofu	6 oz	180	11	11	3	10
Vegetable chow mein	8 oz	330	11	48	4	10
Rice	...	...	.	.	.	.
Fried rice w/vegetables	8 oz	390	12	61	2	9
Steamed rice	8 oz	330	1	74	2	7
Appetizers	...	...	.	.	.	.
Fried shrimp	6 piece	260	12	26	Tr	12

FAST FOOD RESTAURANT: (See other Foods and Beverages listed separately)	Serving Size	Cal-ories	Fat (g)	Carb (g)	Fi-ber (g)	Pro-tein (g)
Chicken egg roll	1	190	8	21	3	8
Vegetable spring roll	1	80	3	14	1	2
Sauces	...	...	.	.	.	.
Hot mustard sauce	1 svg	18	0	1	0	0
Hot sauce	2 tsp	10	1	2	0	0
Mandarin sauce	2 oz	70	0	16	0	Tr
Sweet & sour sauce	2 oz	60	0	15	0	Tr
Soy sauce	1 Tbsp	16	0	2	0	2
Papa John's Pizza	...	...	.	.	.	.
Original crust pizza, large-14"	...	...	.	.	.	.
Cheese	1 slice	290	10	39	2	12
Pepperoni	1 slice	345	15	39	2	14
Sausage	1 slice	335	14	38	2	14
Sausage, pepperoni & beef	1 slice	405	20	39	2	18
Sausage & pepperoni	1 slice	348	15	38	2	16
Vegetable garden fresh pizza	1 slice	287	9	40	3	12
Works, the works pizza	1 slice	370	16	40	3	17
Specialty pizzas	...	...	.	.	.	.
Alfredo, spinach	1 slice	303	12	37	2	13
Alfredo, vegetable & chicken	1 slice	310	12	37	2	15
Chicken and bacon BBQ	1 slice	370	14	44	2	17
Hawaiian BBQ chicken	1 slice	375	14	46	2	17
Thin crust pizza, large-14"	...	...	.	.	.	.
Cheese	1 slice	240	13	23	1	10
Pepperoni	1 slice	295	18	23	2	12
Sausage	1 slice	303	18	24	2	13
Sausage, pepperoni & beef	1 slice	371	24	24	2	17
Sausage & pepperoni	1 slice	298	18	23	1	13
Vegetable garden fresh pizza	1 slice	228	11	24	2	9
Works, the works pizza	1 slice	315	18	25	2	14
Specialty pizzas	...	...	.	.	.	.
Alfredo, spinach	1 slice	251	15	22	1	10
Alfredo, vegetable & chicken	1 slice	276	15	22	1	14
Chicken and bacon BBQ	1 slice	336	18	30	1	15
Hawaiian BBQ chicken	1 slice	324	17	31	1	14
Side items	...	...	.	.	.	.
BBQ dipping sauce	1 svg	48	0	10	0	0
Bread sticks	1 svg	140	2	26	1	4
Buffalo hot sauce	1 svg	25	1	3	0	0
Cheese sauce	1 svg	60	5	0	0	4

FAST FOOD RESTAURANT: (See other Foods and Beverages listed separately)	Serving Size	Cal-ories	Fat (g)	Carb (g)	Fi-ber (g)	Pro-tein (g)
Cheese sticks	1 svg	180	8	20	1	8
Chicken strips	1 svg	83	4	5	Tr	6
Cinnapie	1 svg	114	6	14	0	1
Garlic sauce	1 svg	235	26	0	0	0
Honey mustard dipping sauce	1 svg	190	19	6	0	0
Pizza sauce	1 svg	25	2	3	2	0
Ranch dipping sauce	1 svg	140	14	2	0	1
Pizza Hut	...	...	.	.	.	.
Apple dessert pizza	1 slice	255	5	48	2	3
Bread stick	1	130	4	20	1	3
Bread stick sauce for dipping	1 svg	30	1	5	0	0
Buffalo wings, hot	4	210	12	4	0	22
Buffalo wings, mild	5	200	12	0	0	23
Cavatini pasta	1 svg	485	14	66	9	21
Cavatini pasta supreme	1 svg	565	19	73	10	24
Cherry dessert pizza	1 slice	250	5	47	3	3
Garlic bread	1 slice	150	8	16	1	3
Ham and cheese sandwich	1	555	21	57	4	33
Hand tossed pizza	...	...	.	.	.	.
Beef	1 slice	260	9	16	2	16
Cheese	1 slice	235	7	29	2	12
Ham	1 slice	215	5	28	2	14
Pepperoni	1 slice	238	8	28	2	13
Sausage	1 slice	265	11	28	2	16
Supreme	1 slice	284	12	29	3	13
Pan pizza	...	...	.	.	.	.
Beef	1 slice	285	13	28	2	14
Cheese	1 slice	260	11	28	2	12
Ham	1 slice	240	9	28	2	11
Pepperoni	1 slice	265	12	28	2	11
Supreme	1 slice	310	15	28	3	15
Veggie	1 slice	245	10	29	3	10
Spaghetti with marina sauce	1 svg	490	6	91	8	18
Spaghetti with meat sauce	1 svg	600	13	98	9	23
Spaghetti with meatballs	1 svg	850	24	120	10	37
Stuffed crust pizza	...	...	.	.	.	.
Beef	1 slice	465	22	46	3	23
Cheese	1 slice	445	19	46	3	22
Ham	1 slice	404	22	45	3	24
Pepperoni	1 slice	440	19	45	3	21

FAST FOOD RESTAURANT: (See other Foods and Beverages listed separately)	Serving Size	Cal-ories	Fat (g)	Carb (g)	Fi-ber (g)	Pro-tein (g)
Sausage	1 slice	480	23	46	3	22
Supreme sandwich	1	640	28	62	4	34
Thin & crispy pizza	...	...	.	.	.	.
Beef	1 slice	230	11	22	1	13
Cheese	1 slice	205	8	22	1	10
Ham	1 slice	185	7	21	1	9
Pepperoni	1 slice	215	10	21	1	9
Sausage	1 slice	235	12	22	1	12
Supreme	1 slice	255	13	23	1	12
Veggie	1 slice	185	7	24	2	8
Subway	...	...	.	.	.	.
Six Inch subs	...	...	.	.	.	.
BLT on wheat	1	325	10	44	3	14
BLT on white	1	310	10	38	3	14
Classic Italian BMT wheat	1	460	22	45	3	21
Classic Italian BMT white	1	445	21	39	3	21
Cold cut trio on wheat	1	380	13	46	3	20
Cold cut trio on white	1	360	13	39	3	19
Ham on wheat	1	300	5	45	3	19
Ham on white	1	287	5	39	3	18
Meatball on wheat	1	420	16	51	3	19
Meatball on white	1	405	16	44	3	18
Pizza sub wheat	1	465	22	48	3	19
Pizza sub white	1	448	22	41	3	19
Roast beef on wheat	1	305	5	45	3	20
Roast beef on white	1	288	5	39	3	19
Roasted chicken breast, wheat	1	348	6	47	3	27
Roasted chicken breast, white	1	332	6	41	3	26
Spicy Italian wheat	1	482	25	44	3	21
Spice Italian white	1	465	24	38	3	20
Steak & cheese wheat	1	395	10	47	3	30
Steak & cheese white	1	383	10	41	3	29
Subway club wheat	1	310	5	46	3	21
Subway club white	1	295	5	40	3	21
Subway melt wheat	1	382	12	46	3	23
Subway melt white	1	366	12	40	3	22
Subway seafood & crab, wheat	1	430	19	44	3	20
Subway seafood & crab, white	1	415	19	38	3	19
Tuna on wheat	1	542	32	44	3	19
Tuna on white	1	527	32	38	3	18

FAST FOOD RESTAURANT: (See other Foods and Beverages listed separately)	Serving Size	Cal-ories	Fat (g)	Carb (g)	Fi-ber (g)	Pro-tein (g)
Turkey breast & ham, wheat	1	280	5	39	3	18
Turkey breast & ham, white	1	295	5	46	3	18
Turkey on wheat	1	289	4	46	3	18
Turkey on white	1	273	4	40	3	17
Veggie delite wheat	1	235	3	34	3	9
Veggie delite white	1	220	3	38	3	9
Taco subs	...	...	.	.	.	.
Chicken taco sub wheat	1	436	16	49	4	25
Chicken taco sub white	1	421	16	43	3	24
Beverages	...	...	.	.	.	.
Berry lishus drink	small	113	0	28	1	0
Peach pizazz drink	small	103	0	26	1	0
Pineapple delight drink	small	133	0	33	1	1
Sunrise refresher drink	small	119	0	29	1	1
Cookies	...	...	.	.	.	.
Brazil nut & chocolate chip	1	230	12	27	1	3
Chocolate chip cookie	1	210	10	29	1	2
Chocolate chip, M&M cookie	1	210	10	29	1	2
Chocolate chunk cookie	1	210	10	29	1	2
Oatmeal raisin cookie	1	205	8	29	1	3
Peanut butter cookie	1	220	12	26	1	3
Sugar cookie	1	230	12	28	0	2
White chip macadamia nut	1	235	12	28	0	2
Taco Bell	...	...	.	.	.	.
Bacon cheeseburger	1	565	30	43	4	29
Bean burrito	1	378	12	55	12	13
Big beef meximelt	1	300	16	21	2	16
Big beef nachos supreme	1	435	24	43	9	12
Big beef supreme	1	518	23	52	9	26
Breakfast cheese quesadilla	1	390	22	32	1	0
Breakfast quesadilla with bacon	1	465	28	33	1	1
Breakfast quesadilla w/ sausage	1	440	26	33	1	0
Burrito supreme	1	440	18	50	8	19
Cheddar cheese	1 svg	30	2	0	0	2
Cheese quesadilla	1	370	20	32	1	16
Chicken club	1	540	31	43	4	22
Chicken fajita	1	460	21	49	3	18
Chicken fajita supreme	1	500	25	51	3	19
Chicken quesadilla	1	420	22	33	1	24

FAST FOOD RESTAURANT: (See other Foods and Beverages listed separately)	Serving Size	Cal-ories	Fat (g)	Carb (g)	Fi-ber (g)	Pro-tein (g)
Chili with cheese	1 svg	330	13	43	4	22
Cinnamon twists	1 svg	140	6	19	0	1
Country burrito	1	270	14	26	1	1
Double bacon & egg burrito	1	480	27	39	2	2
Double decker supreme	1	390	18	39	8	16
Double decker taco	1	340	15	37	8	16
Fiesta burrito	1	280	16	25	1	1
Grande burrito	1	420	22	43	2	2
Green sauce	1 svg	5	0	1	0	0
Guacamole	1 svg	35	3	2	1	0
Hot taco sauce	1 svg	0	0	0	0	0
Kid's soft taco roll-up	1	290	16	20	2	16
Light chicken	1	310	8	41	3	18
Light chicken soft taco	1	180	5	21	2	13
Light chicken supreme	1	430	13	52	3	25
Light kid's chicken soft taco	1	180	5	20	1	13
Mexican pizza	1	570	36	41	6	21
Mexican rice	1 svg	190	10	20	0	6
Mild taco sauce	1 svg	0	0	0	0	0
Nacho cheese sauce	1 svg	120	10	5	0	2
Nachos	1	315	18	34	3	2
Nachos belle grande	1	740	39	83	17	16
Pepper jack cheese	1 svg	25	2	1	0	0
Picante sauce	1 svg	0	0	1	0	0
Pinto & cheese	1	195	8	18	10	9
Red sauce	1 svg	10	0	2	0	0
Salsa	1 svg	25	0	5	0	1
Seven layer burrito	1	540	24	65	14	16
Soft taco	1	210	10	20	2	12
Soft taco, BLT	1	340	23	22	2	11
Soft taco, steak	1	510	25	50	3	21
Steak fajita	1	465	21	49	3	18
Taco, hard shell	1	200	7	18	1	14
Taco salad	1	170	10	11	1	10
Taco salad with salsa w/o shell	1	420	21	29	13	26
Taco supreme	1	260	14	22	2	13
Tostada	1	305	14	31	11	11
Veggie fajita	1	420	19	51	3	11
Veggie fajita supreme	1	465	23	53	3	11

FAST FOOD RESTAURANT: (See other Foods and Beverages listed separately)	Serving Size	Cal-ories	Fat (g)	Carb (g)	Fi-ber (g)	Pro-tein (g)
Wendy's	...	...	.	.	.	.
Baked potato w/ bacon & cheese	1	535	18	78	3	17
Baked potato w/ broccoli, cheese	1	470	14	80	3	9
Baked potato with cheese	1	570	23	78	3	14
Baked potato w/ chili & cheese	1	625	24	83	3	20
Baked potato, sour cream, chive	1	370	5	73	3	7
Big bacon classic hamburger	1	640	36	44	2	37
Breaded chicken fillet	1	220	10	11	2	21
Breaded chicken sandwich	1	450	20	43	2	16
Caesar salad	1	110	6	6	2	9
Cheeseburger kids' meal	1	310	13	33	2	187
Chicken Caesar pita	1	485	19	48	2	30
Chicken club sandwich	1	520	25	44	3	30
Chicken nuggets, 5 per svg	1 svg	190	13	9	2	9
Chili (large)	1 svg	310	10	32	1	23
Chili (small)	1 svg	210	7	21	1	15
Chocolate chip cookie	1	270	11	38	1	4
Classic Greek pita	1	440	20	50	1	16
Classic hamburger, single	1	360	16	45	1	24
Classic hamburger w/ everything	1	420	20	31	2	25
Coleslaw	1 svg	45	3	5	1	0
French fries (biggie)	1	470	23	61	4	7
French fries (small)	1	270	13	35	2	4
French fries (super)	1	570	27	73	5	8
Frosty (large)	1	570	17	95	5	15
Frosty (medium)	1	460	13	76	4	12
Frosty (small)	1	340	10	57	3	9
Garden ranch chicken pita	1	480	18	51	2	27
Garden veggie pita	1	400	17	52	3	11
Grilled chicken fillet, w/o bun	1	100	3	0	0	19
Grilled chicken salad	1	190	8	10	2	22
Grilled chicken sandwich	1	290	7	35	2	24
Hamburger kids' meal	1	270	9	33	2	15
Junior bacon cheeseburger	1	445	25	33	2	22
Junior cheeseburger	1	320	13	34	2	18
Junior cheeseburger deluxe	1	360	17	36	2	18
Junior hamburger	1	270	9	34	2	15
Kaiser bun	1	190	3	36	2	6
Sandwich bun	1	160	3	29	2	5
Spicy chicken sandwich	1	415	15	43	3	28
Strawberry banana dessert	1	30	0	8	1	Tr

FAST FOOD RESTAURANT: (See other Foods and Beverages listed separately)	Serving Size	Cal- ories	Fat (g)	Carb (g)	Fi- ber (g)	Pro- tein (g)
Taco salad	1	375	19	28	1	26
White Castle	....	...	.	.	.	.
Breakfast sandwich, regular	1	335	25	17	1	14
Cheeseburger	1	235	14	11	1	7
Cheeseburger with bacon	1	200	13	12	1	10
Cheeseburger, double	1	285	18	12	1	14
Cheesesticks, 5 per svg	1 svg	490	28	32	1	25
Chicken rings, 6 per svg	1 svg	310	21	17	2	16
Chicken ring sandwich	1	170	7	15	2	5
Chocolate shake	14 oz	220	7	32	1	8
Fish sandwich	1	160	6	18	1	8
French fries, small	1	115	6	15	1	1
Hamburger	1	135	7	11	1	6
Hamburger, double	1	235	14	16	1	11
Onion rings, 8 per svg	1 svg	455	25	45	1	12
Vanilla shake	14 oz	228	7	35	0	8

Do you want to know the secrets to safe, easy, effective, and permanent results in managing your weight? Do you want to enjoy a lifetime of optimal health at your perfect weight? If so, this book is for you. Inside, find the power & the knowledge to control your weight forever!

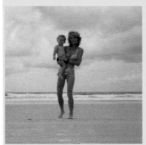

This Mom is Fit at 40! Learn the Secrets!

First, you need a fast & easy to use calorie & nutrient counter to help you make smart food choices. Whether you are a pro, or a novice at counting calories, you will find this book contains all the data you need for fast, easy, accurate food counts. Experts agree calories count first in weight management. The EZ! Fitness Diet & Exercise Guide is included to help you shape and tone your body, and achieve optimal health while maintaining your ideal weight! This book contains the two essential tools for easy lifetime weight management.

Inside find all the foods you love to eat. All the most popular and most common foods, fast food restaurants, brand names, beverages, and alcohol. About 3,500 listings included.

Slim sized to fit in your purse or briefcase. Use it at home, and carry it wherever you go. You can trust the information from this author; a professional licensed healthcare therapist and medical writer.

3386393

Made in the USA